Caring for Self

Other Redleaf Press books by Ingrid Anderson
With Jean Barbre

Supporting Children's Mental Health and Wellbeing: A Strength-Based Approach for Early Childhood Educators

Caring for Self

A Workbook for Early Childhood Educator Well-Being

Jennifer J. Baumgartner, PhD, and
Ingrid Mari Anderson, EdD

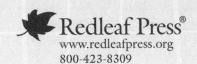
Redleaf Press®
www.redleafpress.org
800-423-8309

Published by Redleaf Press
10 Yorkton Court
St. Paul, MN 55117
www.redleafpress.org

First edition 2024
Cover design by Jesse Hughes
Cover photographs by Jacob Lund; candy1812; H_Ko; Johnér/stock.adobe.com
Interior design by Wendy Holdman
Typeset in Calluna
Printed in the United States of America
31 30 29 28 27 26 25 24   1 2 3 4 5 6 7 8

Library of Congress Cataloging-in-Publication Data

Names: Baumgartner, Jennifer J., author. | Anderson, Ingrid Mari, 1967- author.
Title: Caring for self : a workbook for early childhood educator well-being /
    by Jennifer J. Baumgartner, PhD, and Ingrid Mari Anderson, EdD.
Description: First edition. | St. Paul, MN : Redleaf Press, [2024] | Includes bibliographical references. |
    Summary: "This book supports early childhood educators in addressing the complexities of
    their health-emotional, physical, cognitive, and social-in the increasingly complex and changing
    landscape of early childhood. With reflective practice prompts and activities, it shines a light
    on the emotional work of teaching and caring for young children while teaching skills to help
    burnout and compassion fatigue through resiliency practices and true self-care"—Provided by
    publisher.
Identifiers: LCCN 2023039584 (print) | LCCN 2023039585 (ebook) |
    ISBN 9781605547855 (paperback) | ISBN 9781605547862 (ebook)
Subjects: LCSH: Early childhood educators—Mental health. | Early childhood educators—
    Professional relationships. | Early childhood educators—Job stress—Prevention. | Early childhood
    education—Psychological aspects.
Classification: LCC LB1775.6 .B38 2024 (print) | LCC LB1775.6 (ebook) |
    DDC 372.2101/9—dc23/eng/20230913
LC record available at https://lccn.loc.gov/2023039584
LC ebook record available at https://lccn.loc.gov/2023039585

Printed on acid-free paper

To Wade, Abby, Anna, and James, who support, encourage, and remind me to embrace detours with joy.
    —Jenny

To Greg, who has stood by me in this journey and every journey. Your dedication to our shared profession and decades-long passion for well-being centers me every day. You are my heart.
    —Ingrid

Contents

Acknowledgments

O ur own well-being would look significantly different if not for the support of Melissa York, our Redleaf Press editor and thought partner on this journey. Thank you, Melissa, for nudging us and encouraging all the drafts of the workbook until we had clarity of thought. Your guidance helped us find our way. We would also like to thank Jesse Hughes for the cover that captured our ideas with such vibrancy, as well as Wendy Holdman, who created the final formatting and graphic design of this workbook. Thank you to managing editor Douglas Schmitz for supporting us in all the final steps of the process to help us publish a book supporting early childhood educators' well-being.

We want to thank the students who started this journey with us in our winter 2021 class on self-care and well-being at Portland State University. We thank all the early childhood educators and home visitors who were courageous in their vulnerability, sharing stories of struggles and successes and the work it takes to hold on to oneself while being fully present in the lives of young children and their families.

In addition, Ingrid would like to thank her colleagues, including Sally Guyon, Jean Barbre, Lynn Green, and Vanessa Rodriguez, who provide encouragement and thoughtful reflection and whose practice and research inspire her. She offers a special thank-you to Yondella Hall, who—in sharing her story—has made a profound impact on Ingrid's life by demonstrating the importance of relational well-being, where we are all authentically seen and heard.

Jenny would like to thank her colleagues Russell Carson, Cynthia DiCarlo, and Carrie Ota, who have influenced her thinking about early childhood educators' well-being. She gives thanks to her mentors and exceptional university teachers and leaders, including Jacqueline Bach, Hillary Eisworth, and Marybeth Lima, who encourage and inspire the continual pursuit of excellence. She thanks the Louisiana State University's Communication across the Curriculum team, which generously gave Jenny time and space for this project. And finally, she gives special thanks to the Fred Rogers Institute, the Educators' Neighborhood, and the 2023 cohort of Inquiry Educators for the conversations and sharing that help her remember the "why."

Finally, we would both like to express our appreciation for the National Association of Early Childhood Teacher Educators (NAECTE). In the spring of 2020, and in the midst of a global pandemic, the virtual conference brought us together. An initial connection led to nearly weekly meetings and a thought and writing partnership that produced articles, conference presentations, coteaching experiences, and this book on the topic of well-being. At the heart of this thought partnership is a friendship that is lasting and true.

Introduction

Stress is no stranger to most of us. *Caring for Self: A Workbook for Early Childhood Educator Well-Being* supports early childhood professionals in building sustainable practices and approaches for the well-being of themselves and their teams. This workbook helps early childhood educators reflect on the meaning, emotions, and professional skills of self-stewardship in caring for themselves. We will walk through steps of reflection, address the **emotional work** of identifying and accessing supports, and develop professional skills in the pursuit of well-being. There are many books on reflective practices and how to do the work in early childhood education, but this workbook differs by focusing on the skills necessary to navigate the *emotions* of the work while pursuing well-being. In this workbook, the *skills* are grounded in reflective practices to support your well-being. These are different from the skills we might learn as we prepare to work with children.

As teachers, we rightfully spend a lot of time thinking about "what we do." In these pages, we invite you to explore "who you are." Well-being emerges from understanding who we are and how we care for ourselves. In order to do this, we must spend time noticing how we engage in reflective practices, emotional work, and professional skills development, which together create a pathway to sustainable well-being practices.

- *Reflective practices* are the personal and professional actions we take to understand ourselves. In this workbook, we will begin reflections with a time of *noticing*. When we practice noticing, we want to encourage you to focus on what you see and sense and know, as well as the judgments that come up, without jumping to conclusions.
- *Emotional work* refers to the process of identifying, accessing, and applying tools to navigate emotions and build relationships that support our well-being. While we look at physical, emotional, cognitive, social, psychological, and spiritual dimensions of our work, we focus on our emotions. Our **emotional health** is at the foundation of well-being, so many of our activities will involve noticing our emotions.
- *Professional skills* help us navigate the "how-to" of our work. There are many books that cover the professional competencies we need to understand children's development, support their learning, and guide their behaviors. These skills can play a role in supporting teacher well-being (Jeon, Buettner, and Grant 2018). In this workbook, we focus on skills connected to our identity, our ability to access supports and work with people, and our capacity to solve problems.

1

This workbook is divided into three sections, each focused on the pursuit of well-being.

Part 1: Well-Being: Reflecting on Care of Self. In this first section, we establish the framework for well-being. Chapter 1 considers the whole self: physical, emotional, cognitive, social, psychological, and spiritual. It looks at models of well-being and explores why well-being should be important to us. Chapter 2 discusses our sense of well-being and how we evaluate our well-being. Chapter 3 looks at stress as a potential threat to well-being.

Part 2: Self-Stewardship: Making Choices That Protect Our Well-Being. In this section, we emphasize self-stewardship as the heart of caring for ourselves by making decisions that support our well-being. In chapter 4, we introduce self-stewardship as a practice to navigate well-being, while in chapter 5, we identify barriers to self-stewardship.

Part 3: Professional Skills: Filling Our Toolboxes. In the final section of the book, we aim to fill our toolboxes with resources for our work. We start in chapter 6 by developing a strong professional identity. Chapter 7 focuses on identifying and accessing resources for our emotional work, and chapter 8 builds our interpersonal professional skills. Chapter 9 looks at how we solve problems every day, and chapter 10 summarizes what we've learned with the Problem-Solving Pathway.

Within each section, activities focus on our professional selves. We acknowledge that our work in early childhood intertwines both who we are and what we do, so some activities connect with our personal selves too. Activities that focus on our personal selves help us identify how our experiences, histories, values, and beliefs all influence us as professionals. Reflections on who we are as professionals help us establish or reinforce healthy practices, including clarifying our professional values, determining professional boundaries, solving problems, and establishing a professional reflective practice. In supporting early childhood educators in doing this work, we have discovered that our sense of self and understanding of self-care evolve. You may find it helpful to document this experience, so we have included prompts and a graphic organizer at the close of each chapter that ask you to reflect on your learning.

Why We Wrote This Book

We, Ingrid and Jenny, have each worked in early childhood education for decades, engaging with students and both new and experienced early childhood educators. When we met at a professional conference, our conversation quickly turned to an issue we each care about deeply—the well-being of early childhood teachers. Since 2020 we have been thinking, writing, and publishing on this topic.

Ingrid has been an early childhood teacher, director, multisite coordinator, administrator, college faculty member, and researcher. She has worked in early childhood in nonprofit, school district, and city government early childhood programs; in administration with county and state agencies; and as a faculty member at community colleges and universities in the United States and abroad. She works with programs across the United States and in Italy, Peru, Singapore, and China, always focused on the emotional lives of early childhood educators.

Jenny came to the early childhood profession through early childhood laboratory schools. As a classroom assistant, researcher, director, and now college instructor, she has consistently considered the stories and perspectives of early childhood teachers in her work. Her research on stress and coping in child care and other early childhood settings seeks to acknowledge and equip teachers in their important work while giving voice to their experiences, struggles, and unique expertise.

How to Use This Workbook

This is a workbook and we hope that you will use it in the way that feels comfortable to you. Write and mark in the book, add stickies and notes, draw and doodle. We know not everyone loves to write, so do what is comfortable for you—draw, doodle, outline—it all works. Consider this book and us, the authors, as partners on your wellness journey. It can be tempting to skip over this, but we invite you to take the time to fill in these spaces provided and capture your experiences, discoveries, and reflections. In addition to the text, each chapter is organized into four essential questions, activities to explore well-being and close-of-chapter reflections. You will find spaces to put down your thoughts. This is your space, your time, and your opportunity to embrace well-being. So pick up that pen, pencil, crayon, marker and start your journey.

PART 1

Well-Being: Reflecting on Care of Self

You are setting up the environment for tomorrow. The children are interested in three big ideas. You have room to set up two activities that build on the children's interests. What do you choose?

Sara bites when anyone takes her toy. One parent asks, "Is there a three-bite penalty, and then the child is asked to leave?" You know why young children bite. You are working with Sara to support nonbiting actions in the classroom. But that does not change your worry every time she bites. How do you help Sara and balance other parents' expectations?

A coteacher made a decision in the classroom that concerns you and that you disagree with. You know that you need to approach her. The only time to do so is during your brief lunch break or at the end of the day. How do you communicate your concerns and take the break you need?

You have a licensing visit coming up at your center. Your director is a little nervous. She just came by your room, asking you to stay late tonight. You have someplace you need to be right after work. How do you communicate with your director about how that request affects you?

In the early childhood field, we face problems like those described in the above scenarios every day. Working in early childhood education is complex and involves not only professional skills but also reflective practices and emotional work. Our work in early childhood is complex. We center our well-being by attending to our emotional health.

In part 1, we develop definitions and descriptions for well-being and what it means to each of us. We come to understand the dimensions of well-being, looking at the whole self. Well-being is personal and essential for our emotional health. We learn that we must focus on our own well-being in self-care to be healthy and whole. Well-being is more than the physical self. It also involves our emotional, cognitive, social, psychological, and spiritual selves. We explore self-compassion as a component of caring for self and learn to recognize the stressors of early childhood that affect our well-being. Understanding the role **stress** plays in our lives helps us create **coping** strategies to attend to our emotional health. All of this prepares us to center on self-stewardship as a practice and to build professional skills that fill our toolboxes.

CHAPTER 1

What Is Well-Being?

Well-being is a positive sense of self that allows individuals to lead happy, productive lives and form and maintain healthy relationships.

We celebrate well-being as essential to a fulfilling life. For many of us, lessons about how to be well started in our early childhood years when adults in our lives taught us the importance of eating enough food, getting rest, moving our bodies, and so on. For some, these lessons about **physical well-being** were complemented with skills in handling emotions and social interactions. From these early lessons, we live our lives, pursuing happiness and productivity. But there are moments when the concept of "being well" takes on new meaning. During the COVID-19 pandemic, "be well" was a common farewell when leaving a phone or video conversation. And in this message, we often meant more than "be well from illness" or "stay healthy." Instead, "well" recognized the many parts of being, the ***whole self***: physical, emotional, cognitive, social, psychological, and spiritual. During this time when our regular routines were interrupted, our shared value of well-being came front and center.

In this chapter, we will explore the meaning of well-being—what it is and why it is important. We ask the following questions:

- How is well-being holistic?
- Why does well-being need to be individualized?
- Why is well-being essential?
- Why is well-being important to us?

The study of well-being overlaps with the concept of ***wellness***. Because well-being is generally used to reference all aspects of self, we have chosen to use this word throughout the book. However, it is important to note that pursuing well-being requires wellness, which is defined as "an active process through which people become aware of, and make choices toward, a more successful existence" (National Wellness Institute n.d.).

The Relationship between Wellness and Well-Being

Using the graphic below, reflect on what you see as the relationship between wellness and well-being. We have left a space for you to write.

Wellness is the active process of making choices toward well-being.

Well-being is the outcome of wellness.

Now let us dig a little deeper into the meaning of well-being. In this book, we describe well-being as *holistic (whole person), personal,* and *essential.* Let us explore each of these.

Well-Being Is Holistic

Early childhood educators like to talk about teaching the *whole child*. This idea is a foundational principle in NAEYC's *Developmentally Appropriate Practice,* which encompasses decades of research on domains of human development (NAEYC 2022). These domains are intertwined and support one another. In other words, healthy development of an individual is best achieved when all domains are supported. While researchers and theorists vary in the number of categories and terms they use to describe these "parts of self" or *domains*, six are commonly mentioned:

- physical
- emotional
- cognitive
- social
- psychological
- spiritual

The domains of development hold true for adults as well as children, and perhaps it is unsurprising that multiple theories and approaches to the study of wellness and well-being focus on similar domains. Beginning with a review of some of the most common frameworks for wellness can give us a language and a foundation for our later discussions of well-being. Regardless of the model of wellness adopted, well-being includes multiple domains, is personal and unique to each of us and is essential for our life. We are drawing on research, but there are many factors that affect well-being—individual experiences, cultural and societal norms, and environmental factors, to name a few. The following are several models of wellness.

Indivisible Self Model of Wellness

Jane Myers and Thomas Sweeney (2004), both counseling psychologists, studied how all parts of ourselves are connected together. Rather than segmenting our identity into parts, such as the professional self, spiritual self, or family self, they believe that all parts of ourselves are integrated and interconnected. Myers and Sweeney identify this integration as the *indivisible self* and state that wellness can be achieved only when all aspects (creative, coping, social, essential, physical) of a person are well. The theory of the *indivisible self* highlights how all dimensions of ourselves are integrated; therefore, well-being practices also need to be integrated, connecting all aspects of ourselves. As we work on building a sustainable approach to well-being, it is imperative to think about how we nurture, utilize, and build on holistic practices. If we neglect one area of our well-being, then other areas will be out of balance.

Dimensions of Wellness Models

There are several models of wellness based on the premise that wellness is interconnected and holistic. These models focus on five to eight dimensions. The National Institute of Wellness (Hettler 1976) developed six dimensions of wellness for healthy living: emotional, environmental, intellectual, physical, social, and spiritual wellness. While the eight-dimensional model (J. Flowers Health Institute n.d.) adds occupational and financial wellness to the six, the five-dimensional one (Rath and Harter 2010) focuses on career, social, financial, physical, and community well-being. All models focus on areas of life that contribute to our overall wellness.

Dimensions of wellness are used in research to measure how healthy individuals are in each category. However, we need to acknowledge that there are systemic barriers that create uneven and sometimes inaccurate measurements of well-being. These dimensions of wellness models do not necessarily account for cultural measurements of well-being.

Considering Culture in Well-Being

Tara Yosso (2005) studied cultural wealth as a form of human capital that is deeply rooted in experiences and histories in communities of color. Environmental and historical trauma such as colonization, displacement, boarding schools, and genocide all impact generational well-being, scaffolding the understanding that well-being is shaped not only by the individual but in the context of the broader society.

Well-being in a cultural context considers communities and their cultural wealth, which is made up of their cultural knowledges (often generational), skills, and practices. Religious or spiritual practices and traditions are all part of cultural wealth, as well as traditional foods, medicines, and healing practices.

Cultural models of well-being employ strength-based approaches that build cultural capital and center identity, language use, and connections to the community. Cultural well-being models include families, communities, and social networks (often developed over generations) in navigating social and economic injustices. They support individuals and communities in addressing discrimination and stigma.

Well-Being Is Personal

Well-being means something different to each person and is shaped by our individual identities, including our personal experiences, beliefs, values, and contexts. Culture plays a central role in who we are and how we navigate the world, and so well-being depends on the context of our individual and community cultures. We started this chapter with a definition of *well-being*; look at it again and think about how you might add to the definition so that it reflects your own ideas.

Well-being: a positive sense of self that allows individuals to lead happy, productive lives and form and maintain healthy relationships.

Each of us comes to our well-being practice with a different lens. In other words, the way each of us defines *happy* and *productive* is different based on our experiences, values, and contexts. Take a minute and go back to the definition of well-being. Underline the words that you need to understand for yourself before moving forward. As we begin to think about well-being, start considering your own definition of these things.

Defining Well-Being

Write your own definition below for each of the words included in the definition of well-being. How do each look for you?

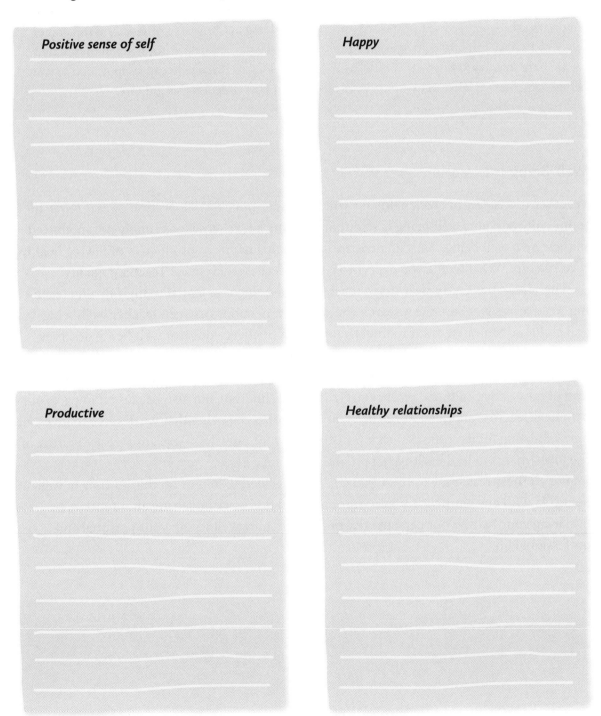

Positive sense of self

Happy

Productive

Healthy relationships

You Are Worthy of Well-Being

Being well is becoming a lost art in the modern world. As early childhood professionals, our own needs are often subjugated by the **demands** placed on us. Our profession speaks of well-being as something that we do for the children's sake—we need to take care of ourselves so that we can take care of others. But we are here to encourage you to look at well-being from another lens. You are worthy of being well and being in care of yourself. Period. No justifications are needed. Each of your journeys will be unique. On the many paths to well-being, practice **self-compassion** and care of self. Be attentive to your needs while holding awareness of others. And remember that well-being does not happen in isolation, so look to those who can support you as you support them on this journey.

Well-Being Is Essential

Whether it was easy or challenging for you to develop your own definition of *well-being*, intentionally pursuing well-being is essential. Imagine a teacher who is simply not interested in their own well-being. They do not care about being happy or productive or having healthy relationships. What would you expect to be the effect on their lives? Teaching quality?

The research is pretty clear that a teacher's well-being is essential to high-quality teaching. Yet even as we share the research about the connections between teacher well-being and child outcomes, we want to underscore that we believe educator well-being deserves focus for its own sake. It matters not just because our **emotional health** and well-being impact the children in our classrooms and schools (see de Schipper et al. 2009 for exploration of how early childhood teacher stress impacts children), but also because it impacts our own health across our lives. At the heart of this book is the belief that we deserve to invest in our well-being for its own sake—not for others, but for ourselves—because we are worthy of the investments to lead healthy, happy, and productive lives.

For all these reasons, we are so glad you have decided to join us on this journey to well-being. As with any journey, it is important to begin this work by setting an intention, or declaring your "why," your personal reason, for pursuing wellness in your personal and professional life.

Why Is Well-Being Important to You?

It is also important to note that the concept of caring for self varies across cultures. While some define self-care as an individualized practice, others see self-care as a collective action embedded in their community.

Why do you see well-being as important?

Why do you need well-being?

Why are you worthy of well-being?

Why is well-being a priority to you right now?

You will come back to your "why" over and over again throughout this process, especially when things are hard or when you feel compelled to prioritize others' asks at the expense of your own needs.

Reflection on Practice

At the end of each chapter, you will find our questions from the beginning of the chapter to reflect and write on here. Let's take a moment to notice what was important to us in this chapter.

How is well-being holistic?

Why does well-being need to be individualized?

Why is well-being essential?

Why is well-being important to you?

CHAPTER 2

Well-Being and You

Being in care of self is the ongoing practice of taking responsibility for one's own physical, emotional, cognitive, social, psychological, and spiritual needs through mindful practice.

We must learn to center our own **well-being** and **self-care**. Much like with oxygen masks on a plane, we have to take care of ourselves first—put on our own masks—before we can help others around us. When we are in the care of ourselves, taking responsibility for our own needs, we develop a sense of self-awareness and self-worth while improving our well-being. First, we care for ourselves because we are worthy of care. Second, we care for ourselves to build and sustain meaningful relationships with others. In this chapter, we ask the following questions:

- Why is it important to be proactive in our well-being?
- Why should we be proactive in the care of ourselves?
- What does it mean to balance our well-being?
- Why is self-compassion a valuable practice?

Being Proactive in Our Well-Being

Well-being requires that we practice **being in care of self**, proactively caring for our physical, emotional, cognitive, social, psychological, and spiritual health and well-being. We actively take steps to cultivate habits that benefit our well-being. It is also important to note that the concept of caring for self varies across cultures. While some define self-care as an individualized practice, others see self-care as a collective action embedded in their community. In the Western Eurocentric world today, caring for self or self-care most frequently refers to caring for our physical selves. While physical well-being is a component of caring for self, the more essential parts of well-being include our emotions. It is this essential part that we focus on in this book. We begin by taking a moment to understand our present well-being.

Well-Being and You Survey

How do you care for yourself? In your own notes or in a journal, take stock of your well-being. Answer the questions below by scoring how you feel in your personal and professional life from low to high.

	PERSONAL LIFE		PROFESSIONAL LIFE	
	LOW HIGH		LOW HIGH	
Do I have someone to talk with about my emotions?	1 2 3 4 5		1 2 3 4 5	
Can I say no when I need to?	1 2 3 4 5		1 2 3 4 5	
Am I content most of the time?	1 2 3 4 5		1 2 3 4 5	
Do I have a strong support system to help me through life?	1 2 3 4 5		1 2 3 4 5	
Am I able to relax?	1 2 3 4 5		1 2 3 4 5	
Do I feel proud of who I am or who I am becoming?	1 2 3 4 5		1 2 3 4 5	
Do I see stress as something I can learn from or something to avoid?	1 2 3 4 5		1 2 3 4 5	
Am I aware of bodily sensations, emotions, and behaviors when I am stressed?	1 2 3 4 5		1 2 3 4 5	
Do I allow myself to experience emotions just as they are?	1 2 3 4 5		1 2 3 4 5	
Am I able to care for myself on a daily basis?	1 2 3 4 5		1 2 3 4 5	
Am I able to ask for help when I need it?	1 2 3 4 5		1 2 3 4 5	

adapted from Emotional Wellness checklist

https://www
.unh.edu/health
/emotional-wellness

After you answer these questions, take a few moments to review them and reflect. We encourage you to resist the temptation to assign meaning or build a to-do list. Instead, take a moment to notice which areas are high and which are low. Which areas of your emotional health are very strong (high score)? In what areas might you need more support (low score)? There are no right or wrong scores, and there is no perfect response. Rather, this activity is a starting point for reflecting on areas where you might wish to focus.

Caring for Ourselves and Others

Well-being requires that we practice self-care, proactively caring for our physical, emotional, cognitive, social, psychological, and spiritual health and well-being. When you hear the term *self-care*, you might think of vacations, days off, time to rest, exercise, or massages and manicures. Media and advertisers are quick to promote the concept to sell any number of products and experiences. However, this popular notion of self-care as a break from reality is inconsistent with a healthy practice. It is true that we all need some time away for rest and relaxation, but well-being is much more comprehensive. It goes beyond self-soothing (think of a warm bath or piece of chocolate) and changes our practices and decision-making. Caring for self is about making choices that support us in becoming our best selves.

Caring for ourselves is not selfish, but self-care has come to be viewed as self-serving. For some educators, taking care of ourselves feels uncomfortable at first. As individuals who work in a helping profession, our focus and sense of success are tied to caring for others. The needs (and therefore the demands) of the children and families we serve are seemingly endless. Being professional also means engaging in professional activities, such as professional development and caring for colleagues. Additionally, many early childhood programs lack sufficient **resources**, including people, funding, or time. In this context, the never-ending requests may mean making sacrifices, such as working without breaks, coming in for extra hours, canceling vacations, or skipping time off, to name a few. Many who work in early childhood accept these responsibilities because of their professional commitment to children.

Self-care is about valuing ourselves enough to make choices that renew our emotional health. It is also important in the practice of caring for ourselves that we do not harm others or deplete them in our practice of restoring our own well-being. For example, we may be upset with a colleague. To deal with our emotions, we might complain about this individual to another colleague. While we might temporarily feel better sharing our emotions, the act of complaining is causing harm. Strong self-care actions would be to acknowledge the emotions we have of being upset or angry and to work to address the issue with our colleague and not a third party.

We need to be healthy and whole, and so do our colleagues. When our colleagues are well and whole, then the work we do together is better. Being part of a community means supporting one another in our professional practices with actions such as these:

- **Being Aware**—we work to notice our own states of mind and those of others.
- **Modeling Care of Self**—we prioritize self-care actions within a professional context and ask others to do the same.
- **Mentoring** (formal/informal)—we are transparent in the actions that we take for our own well-being and support others to do the same.

- **Advocating**—we champion practices and policies in the workplace that center well-being.
- **Reflecting**—we are thoughtful about our personal and professional actions and seek to understand what we and others say and do.

Caring for Yourself in Community

While caring for yourself, how can you build up both yourself and others? Reflecting on the descriptions above, think about how you can take action in your own practices.

Our care of selves always happens within the context of community. We strive to keep this in mind as we focus on our own well-being.

Balancing Our Well-Being

What does it mean to balance our well-being? We start by looking at the domains of well-being—physical, emotional, cognitive, social, psychological, and spiritual—and making sure that we engage in actions of self-care in all domains.

Physical well-being is often the primary form of wellness discussed in our society. Practices for physical wellness focus on caring for the physical body, including sleep, healthy eating, hydration, personal health (medical and dental care), and personal care. When you are physically unwell, normal tasks become challenging. Especially when this experience is temporary, you may receive compassion from others and allowances at work. Staying physically well is frequently discussed in the media. Commonly referenced activities for physical well-being include balancing physical movement and passivity, choosing healthy foods and beverages, sleeping for the recommended time, and getting regular health checkups.

Emotional well-being focuses on your state of mind and inner life. It includes practices of recognizing, understanding, responding to, and regulating your own emotions. Activities include expressing and receiving expressions of emotions in ways that are healthy for you and others, setting personal boundaries, engaging in positive self-talk, and practicing self-compassion when you make mistakes.

Cognitive well-being focuses on mental flexibility and imagination. It includes practices that engage your thinking outside of work and can include activities such as hobbies (reading or gardening), skills development (learning to play music or fixing your house), or craft- or art-based activities. It can also include visiting new places, attending events (concerts or community celebrations), and engaging in new experiences. Actions include taking regular time in your week to self-select activities that engage your imagination, such as joining a knitting group or visiting a local park.

Social well-being focuses on relationships and the roles they play in your life. Relationships with others are frequently seen as a critical part of wellness. Practices that facilitate positive interactions between you and others include spending time with friends and family and maintaining close relationships with trusted friends from several social circles. Activities include communicating regularly with friends and family through a variety of engagements (in person, on the phone, and electronically), getting involved in multiple groups (work, informal, and organized social groups), and engaging with individuals and groups that care for your health and well-being.

Psychological well-being focuses on holistic and positive approaches to mental health, emphasizing positive emotions, relationships, and personal growth. It includes the practices of examining the beliefs behind your behaviors and actions and understanding that you have the right to meet your personal needs in healthy ways. Activities include practicing reflection and mindfulness, journaling, spending time with yourself without distraction, and meditating.

Spiritual well-being focuses on your ability to discover meaning and purpose in your life. The spiritual self is a part of everyone, regardless of religiosity or spirituality. A sense of **belonging** and purpose are central to your spiritual self. Practices to support spiritual wellness include time for contemplation and reflection. Activities include belonging to a group pursuing similar goals, discovering marvels, and feeling awe at the world.

Now that we have reviewed the different parts of well-being, let us take inventory of our own wellness and well-being using an activity known as the wellness wheel. In this chapter, we focus on your personal well-being. In chapter 6, we'll focus on your professional well-being using a similar model.

ACTIVITY 2.3

The Personal Wellness Wheel

Take a few minutes to read and reflect on each statement. Then return to circle your answer.

Physical Wellness

Y	N	I have sufficient sleep per night (ideally at least seven restful hours).
Y	N	I make healthy eating choices.
Y	N	I drink multiple cups of water a day.
Y	N	I routinely visit a doctor and dentist.
Y	N	I take time for personal care.
Y	N	I exercise regularly.
Y	N	Other: _____

Emotional Wellness

Y	N	I spend time looking inward.
Y	N	I know how to handle my feelings.
Y	N	I set and hold my boundaries.
Y	N	I separate my work life from my home life.

Y	N	I engage in positive self-talk.
Y	N	I practice self-compassion and regularly forgive myself of my mistakes.
Y	N	Other: _____

Cognitive Wellness

Y	N	I have interests outside of work that I engage in at least weekly.
Y	N	I try new activities or visit new places at least monthly.
Y	N	I read (on paper, online, and so on) or research to learn about topics that interest me.
Y	N	I have specific goals for learning new skills.
Y	N	I am generally satisfied with my education.
Y	N	I would describe myself as a lifelong learner.
Y	N	Other: _____

Social Wellness

Y	N	I work to create positive interactions with others.
Y	N	I spend time with friends and family.
Y	N	I have a small circle of friends that I trust and that trust me in return.
Y	N	I talk to friends and family on a regular basis (at least monthly).
Y	N	I engage in at least two different types of social groups.
Y	N	My social interactions build me up.
Y	N	Other: _____

Psychological Wellness

Y	N	I practice being present in the moment and engaged in what is happening.
Y	N	I have a plan for caring for my physical, emotional, social, cognitive, psychological, and spiritual health.
Y	N	I take time during my day for myself, away from distractions.
Y	N	I spend at least two hours of free time a day without using technology or social media.
Y	N	I have choices in my daily life.
Y	N	I have more positive than negative emotions.
Y	N	Other: _____

Spiritual Wellness

Y	N	I have a general sense of balance.
Y	N	I have an overall sense of well-being.
Y	N	I find meaning and purpose in my life.
Y	N	I understand my values, attitudes, and beliefs.
Y	N	I trust others and am able to forgive.
Y	N	I have a sense of connection with the natural world.
Y	N	Other: _____

For each of the questions to which you answered yes, fill in one segment on the wheel in the corresponding category. Now take a few minutes to fill in the wheel. For each yes, fill in a section of the correct segment on the wheel.

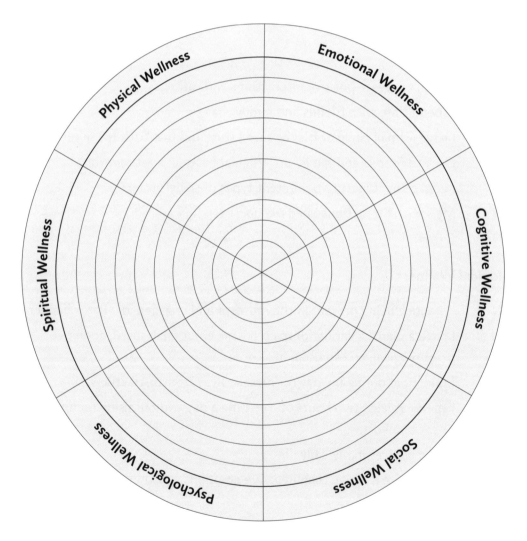

Step back and look at the completed wheel. What areas do you notice as being strong? Which areas are you missing? As you reflect on your wellness in the activity, you may have discovered that you are experiencing a great deal of wellness in some areas of your life but less in other areas. Since each of these domains contributes to your overall well-being, you must spend time building wellness in each and every area. If you are looking for ways to increase your well-being in a domain, go back and look at the statements for ideas. Be careful about creating an action plan or adding to your to-do list too quickly. Remember to treat yourself compassionately as you notice areas for growth or opportunity.

Self-Compassion as a Valuable Practice

We strive to be compassionate with the children in our care by carefully attending to their social and emotional development. We need to attend to our own selves with the same compassion and kindness in our actions, words, and thoughts. When we are kind and loving to ourselves, accepting our flaws and mistakes, we are practicing self-compassion. These actions are not indulgent; rather, they are about acknowledging our common humanity and the fact that we all struggle. With self-compassion, we acknowledge our determined and yet imperfect processes of being the best we can be in our work and in our lives.

ACTIVITY 2.4

What Builds You Up, What Tears You Down

In this activity, think about self-compassion and self-criticism. As you go through your day, what are the messages you tell yourself? Do they build you up? What messages might tear you down? Fill in the figure with some of these messages.

What Builds You Up?
1.
2.
3.
4.
5.

What Tears You Down?
1.
2.
3.
4.
5.

Look back at the messages that tear you down. What can you do to help you resume those messages so they are self-compassionate? Think about language you can use or actions you can take to change the negative to positive and encouraging messages.

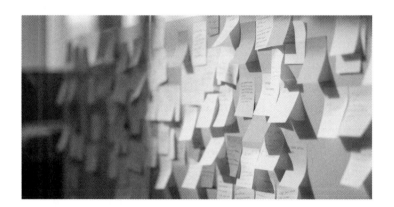

Reflection on Practice

Let's review the questions from the beginning of the chapter.

Why is it important to be proactive in our well-being?

Why should we be proactive in the care of ourselves?

What does it mean to balance our well-being?

Why is self-compassion a valuable practice?

CHAPTER 3

Addressing Stress and Coping as Part of Well-Being

Stress is a natural reaction to demands placed on the body that can come from physically, emotionally, cognitively, psychologically, or spiritually challenging situations.

In chapter 1, we explored the meaning of well-being, including your personal definition and your "why" for pursuing wellness. As we work for well-being, there will undoubtedly be challenges. In this chapter, we will discuss how stress interferes with living happy and productive lives and maintaining healthy relationships. We will explore questions such as these:

- Why is it stressful to work in early childhood?
- How do we define stress?
- What happens when we sustain stress over time?
- How do we cope with our stress?

Working in Early Childhood Can Be Stressful

Our work with young children requires us to be fully present in the classroom, and the structures of our profession require us to be accountable to our programs, parents, licensing requirements, and quality initiatives. While we have autonomy in working with young children in everyday moments, we often do not have control over program structures such as the curriculum, ratios, and licensing and other state and federal requirements.

The tension that arises in having limited control is stressful: we are expected to be autonomous with children and are accountable for children's learning and development, but we have limited control over the larger program structures that surround these processes. This unique environment makes the emotional work required in the early childhood profession different from many other helping professions. The structures of early childhood education are often set up in ways that limit and, in some cases, actively undermine teachers' emotional well-being. Each experience and context is unique. Let's take a moment to consider the stress you experience.

Stressors in Early Childhood Education

Make a list of the things that are stressful for you in the early childhood profession (no matter how big or small).

1. _____

2. _____

3. _____

4. _____

5. _____

6. _____

_____

_____

We will come back to this list later in the chapter. For now, just notice and name the stressors. In this chapter, we will primarily focus on the physical, emotional, cognitive, and social domains. The concepts of psychological and spiritual aspects are deeply intertwined with an individual's unique contexts and are not easily defined in a broad sense. For instance, our psychological reactions are intricately tied to the multifaceted developmental ecosystems that unfold within our unique cultural backgrounds.

Defining Stress

We all experience stress, but what is stress, really? Stress is a **defense response**, a natural re-action to demands placed on the body from physically, mentally, and cognitively challenging situations. Stress can be located in the physical body, or it can be psychological, relational, sociocultural, or personal. Stress is a part of life and can be both positive and negative. Some positive stress motivates us, but negative stress can harm us. A little bit of stress is normal in daily life. Too much stress or long-term stress negatively affects physical and mental health.

Stress is much like the warning signals in our cars. These signals tell us when we need to refuel, change the oil, and check the tire pressure. These little lights can help us know there is a problem before it gets too large (and too expensive). But we have the choice to pay attention to the warnings or to ignore them. Ignoring the fuel gauge may seem like a good response in the moment—when we are in a hurry, when fueling would be inconvenient, or when we don't know where to find the closest gas station. But we put ourselves in jeopardy if we continue to ignore the warning signs.

The Body's Response to Stress Input

Most stress is associated with **somatic symptoms**—that is, you experience the stress physi-cally. For some, this might be butterflies in the stomach that don't leave. Others might experience shortness of breath, stomachaches or headaches, dizziness, or ringing in the ears. It is important to learn your own symptoms and recognize how your body tells you that it is stressed. The strange thing about stress, though, is that it can cause you to lose the ability to notice things. As you work so hard to push through the stress, you may grow accustomed to ignoring the warning signals. And just like the warning signals in a car, ignoring these sig-nals can have big consequences. Research suggests that stress experienced over time leads to poor health, **burnout**, and attrition. Because of the possible and longterm negative impacts of stress, it is important that we pay attention to it. In the next activity, you will have an opportunity to think about some stressors in your life and how you experience them.

Stress and the Body

In this activity, return to the stressors identified in activity 3.1. After reflecting on each stressor, place the stressors in order from high (5) to low (1) below. In the next column, notice how each stressor makes you feel, focusing on the physical or somatic symptoms you experience. Where you do you notice this stress in your body. There is no wrong way to feel stress. What is important is that you start identifying where in your body you feel stress.

MY STRESS LEVEL *Rate from High (5) to Low (1).*	MY STRESSORS	WHERE DO I FEEL THIS STRESS (SOMATIC SYMPTOMS)?
5		
4		
3		
2		
1		

The Brain's Response to Stress

During times of stress, it is not only our bodies that respond with somatic symptoms but also our brains. The brain, which acts as the control center for all sensory input, makes both conscious and unconscious decisions based on the level of stress perceived (see figure 3.1). When the body is highly stressed, the **limbic system** takes over. The limbic system processes basic survival instincts, such as the **fight**-or-**flight** response. Further, it plays an important role in shaping emotions, behaviors, and memories in the unconscious mind. The brain's ability to construct meaning and prescribe appropriate actions (behaviors) based on sensory input and past experience (memories) is crucial for perception (emotions) and understanding the world.

The cerebral cortex is at the center of high-order cognitive functions. It handles high-level cognitive functions, including attention, memory, **problem-solving**, decision-making, and reasoning. The cerebral cortex provides advanced cognitive functioning such as abstract thinking, reasoning, and conscious awareness; it is also responsible for a wide range of

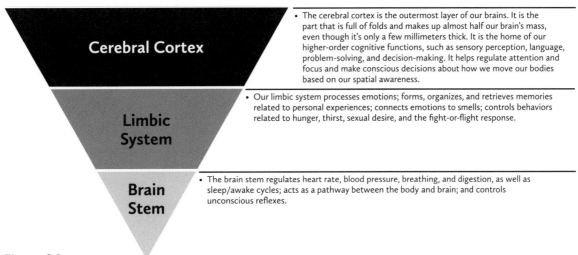

Figure 3.1

complex mental processes and enables us to perceive, think, reason, and interact with our environments. Our emotions are processed in several areas of the brain, including the limbic system and the cerebral cortex. Working together, these areas change our biological and physical states in response to our environments.

Defense Mechanisms for Stress

Our most basic stress responses are to *fight*, *flight*, **freeze**, or **fawn**. The intensity of the response corresponds to how much we feel we are in danger. Psychologist Walter Cannon (1915) first connected the reactions of fight or flight to ancient, ingrained survival instincts or acute stress responses when under threat. Freeze and fawn models emerged to account for threats to our survival that are psychological in nature. All four of these reactions in the modern world are designed to help us deal with threats through a pattern of responses. Fight, flight, freeze, and fawn responses can vary in intensity and include survival instincts in the unconscious brain and conscious processes of defense in our interactions with others. The following graphic shows how fight, flight, freeze, or fawn show up as defense mechanisms in response to stress or perceived threats. Although our fight, flight, freeze, or fawn reactions are typically linked to situations involving severe physical or psychological threats, we frequently observe these behaviors in the context of stress during early childhood experiences. These adapted responses tend to surface as unaddressed stress responses when we try to cope with the emotions we are experiencing. In the subsequent sections of this chapter, we will look at ways we can adapt our coping responses to strength-based approaches that are emotionally healthier for ourselves and those around us.

Fight—using aggressive behaviors to address the threat:
- Physically—using your body, with actions ranging from blocking someone to physically harming them
- Emotionally—talking over others or bullying
- Cognitively—seeing others as competitors or feeling they are against you
- Socially—gossiping, starting rumors, or joking

Flight—getting away from the perceived danger:
- Physically—running from danger
- Emotionally—self-sabotaging or shutting down
- Cognitively—giving in or giving up
- Socially—ignoring or blocking others (such as on social media)

Freeze—being unable to act against a threat:
- Physically—standing in place
- Emotionally—not feeling emotions beyond panic
- Cognitively—struggling with memory or ideas
- Socially—not knowing what to say or do in a situation

Fawn—pleasing others to avoid conflict:
- Physically—putting yourself in place of another, even if it causes harm or discomfort
- Emotionally—saying or believing your needs are less important than others
- Cognitively—rationalizing others' behaviors or actions
- Socially—giving in, doing what others want over what you feel is right

Figure 3.2. Stress coping responses in early childhood settings to physical and psychological threats.

Sustained Stress over Time

Stress responses are triggered when the demands or pressures on our physical and cognitive selves are greater than our ability to cope with them. Regardless of the type or level of stress, all stressors trigger the same pattern of response. The body experiences stress in three stages that look much like an arc.

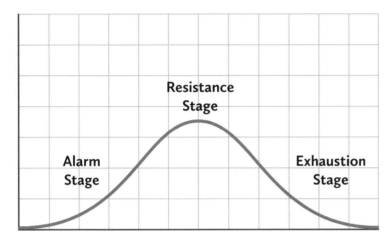

Figure 3.3. Patterns of Stress Responses

Alarm stage—the amygdala is activated and we fight, flee, freeze, or fawn.

Resistance stage—the stress response plateaus, and gradually our heart rate, blood pressure, and elevated body functions decrease as the body moves toward recovery.

Exhaustion stage—when the body continues to experience stress over time, we feel a decrease in overall health. Chronic stress can have long-term health consequences.

When we experience chronic stress, our bodies and brains do not have the important downtime to relax and recover. Without this recovery period, we can experience issues with our physical, social, cognitive, emotional, psychological, and spiritual health.

A Note about Trauma

Before moving on from this discussion of stress as a threat to well-being, we need to explicitly acknowledge the impact of trauma. **Trauma** refers to distressing, disturbing responses following an event or experience that has an adverse effect on one's ability to function. These experiences can be singular, multiple, or repetitive events over time that can occur at any point in our life span. Experiences that are deeply difficult, emotionally challenging or draining, and often repeated continue to have a negative effect on an individual after the event is over.

If we are to pursue wellness, it is critical that we identify traumas and their effects on our own lives. Our reactions to trauma are influenced by our sociocultural history. And our expressions of trauma are as varied as our histories, based on our capacity to navigate our emotions. Attending to trauma is emotionally challenging and best done with support. If you have never had help unpacking a trauma, you might contact a mental health professional. You can also access mental health resources at the National Alliance on Mental Illness or the National Institute of Mental Health linked in the QR codes.

www.nami.org/Home

www.nimh.nih.gov

Coping with Stress

When we experience stress, we look for ways to cope. Coping is what we do to handle or address a challenge or stressor effectively. There are many approaches to coping; some people ignore the issue and avoid addressing negative emotions. Sometimes this looks like ignoring the problem entirely by, for example, ignoring a growing issue with a parent or colleague or just "forgetting" that you need to complete a report. Instead, some people might focus on behaviors that soothe the negative feelings and introduce something positive or pleasurable. Ask any educator and they will likely list several self-soothing approaches that help them get through their days, such as coffee or chocolate. Pushing through the demands and stuffing down emotions may help in the short term, but over time, any coping approaches that ignore a problem and the emotions experienced will ultimately lead to increased stress and risk of burnout.

In order to address our stress from a strength-based approach, we now look at how we can adapt our coping strategies. We need to appraise our stress through evaluation and interpretation. How we perceive stress and determine whether we feel strong enough or have enough resources to cope is critical to our responses. For example, if the intercom interruptions through the day cause you to jump with surprise each time, this may look like stress. But some of us also love being surprised, such as by surprise parties, amusement park rides, and scary movies, just to name a few examples. So, is this the negative kind of stress? Research tells us that it really depends on two things: our thoughts about the event and the skills we have to respond to it.

First, how we perceive, or what researchers call *appraise*, the event has a lot to do with whether it is stressful. When we experience an event, we make many mental decisions to determine whether it represents harm, challenge, threat, or benefit. This first **appraisal** serves as a form of triage (Folkman et al. 1986). This is where we determine if we are in danger. If so, the fight, flight, freeze, or fawn response might be ignited. However, if we perceive that the event is not immediately dangerous, we next think about how we might need to respond: How do we address the present concern? Do we have the ability and resources to handle the current issue? When we have more resources and abilities, we experience less stress (Lazarus and Folkman 1987).

First Appraisal of Stress and Coping

Through this chapter, we define stress and coping as it affects well-being. In this activity, take time to notice and make a first appraisal (or first perception) of those somatic symptoms of stress (or how you feel stress in your body), of your common responses to a stressor or two and then think about them.

Begin thinking about the resources that might help you when you next encounter this stressor.

1. First, look back at activity 3.2, where you identified your stresses and where you felt them in your body.

2. Next, choose one stressor to focus on. Then reflect on the following:

List the Stressor: _____

What do you notice about how you appraise and respond to this stressor?

In the coming chapters we will talk about how we might access resources to help address stress, for now just think about the following.

What would support look like for you as you encounter this stressor?

What Might Help You?	What Skills Might You Need?	What Can Help Your Emotions?

What Did You Notice?

When we work to find supports or resources for addressing stress, we have many choices. Noticing how we might make a connection between coping and identifying resources is part of the first appraisal and one of our first steps in self-stewardship. Throughout the rest of the book, we will continue to build our coping skills as we pursue well-being.

Instead of avoiding a challenge and the emotions involved, healthy coping involves having a clear awareness of the stress and actively choosing a response. There are many ways to do this, but all involve gathering resources, altering demands, or changing how you perceive and feel about the demands and resources, as we will discuss in chapter 5. But first in our next chapter, we will explore more about how make choices to care for ourselves.

Reflection on Practice

At the end of each chapter, you will find our questions from the beginning of the chapter to reflect on here. Let's review the question from the beginning of the chapter.

Why is it stressful to work in early childhood?

How do we define stress?

What happens when we sustain stress over time?

How do we cope with our stress?

PART 2

Self-Stewardship: Making Choices That Protect Our Well-Being

In part 1, we explored the foundations of well-being and developed a definition and description of well-being. We defined well-being as a holistic, personal, and essential part of our personal and professional lives that is necessary for having a positive sense of self, leading a happy and productive life, and maintaining healthy relationships.

At this point of your journey, you likely have a good idea about what well-being means to you. As we move forward together, it will be important to come back to this personal definition to remember what is meaningful, helpful, and soul affirming for you, especially when challenges arise and the pursuit of wellness gets hard.

In this next section, we consider actions and strategies that protect our well-being. Well-being requires us to make choices about how we care for ourselves. Just as the meaning of *being well* is unique for each of us and the challenges to wellness we face and the strategies needed to promoted well-being are specific to individual needs.

Self-stewardship is the process of ensuring our well-being. Part 2 of the book focuses on self-stewardship by examining how we make choices that protect our well-being. Chapter 4 considers self-stewardship and its importance in facing demands. *Demands* are the external pressures or challenges that individuals face in their daily lives, such as work responsibilities, relationship issues, or health problems. Addressing demands effectively by identifying and using the resources we have available is an important part of coping with stress and maintaining well-being. Chapter 5 looks at how we appraise the stress of internal and external demands and how we develop strength-based coping strategies.

Here is an example of demands we face every day:

Maria drives up to the school. Her thoughts are focused on the tasks she must complete before the children arrive in an hour. As she enters the school, she is met at the door by a colleague who needs some help finding manipulatives for her class. Maria stops to locate them in the resource room and, realizing how disordered it has become, makes a mental note to come back to organize it later in the week. Entering the hallway, Maria meets the director, who is walking a new teacher around the school. They stop to talk with Maria, and the director asks if Maria will show the new hire to the break room. Maria agrees and continues the conversation as they walk. After delivering the new teacher to the breakroom and then the correct classroom, Maria's mind swims with the tasks she has to complete, now with less time. She meets a child and parent in the hallway and can tell they have something to discuss with her.

In Maria's story, we see some of the many demands that impact our lives in the classroom. When we lack the resources we need or misidentify the demands, our stress levels can rise. Building self-stewardship begins when we embark on a journey to accurately appraise our emotions and the resources we require to do the work as early childhood educators.

CHAPTER 4

Defining Self-Stewardship

Self-stewardship is the ability to lead one's physical, emotional, cognitive, social, psychological, and spiritual self in ways that actively promote and sustain one's well-being.

These days, stewardship and conservation are hot topics of conversation. As a society, we are learning more each day about the importance of caring for our environment and working toward sustainability. We can take these ideas and apply them to our own self-stewardship. Personal conservation, or what we call *self-stewardship*, addresses the need to care for ourselves and our environments and to engage in processes, routines, and approaches that promote and sustain well-being. We practice self-stewardship because no one can do the work to protect our own well-being except us. In this chapter, we ask questions such as these:

- What is self-stewardship?
- How do we practice self-stewardship?
- Why center ethics and boundaries in our work?
- How do we build strong professional boundaries?

Understanding Self-Stewardship

Caring for anything requires actions, routines, and tools to sustain and support excellence. While frequently applied to caring for a budget, physical space (like a home or garden), or community, the idea of stewardship is helpful when thinking about the activities, approaches, and strategies that promote well-being. There is a difference between caring for something and being a steward. The first involves basic tasks, such as general maintenance, but often with no goal or overall plan. Stewardship requires a proactive and complex understanding of the goals of care.

BEING IN CARE OF SELF IS . . .	SELF-STEWARDSHIP IS . . .
• taking everyday actions that are centered on immediate needs and basic well-being • caring for basic physical, social, emotional, cognitive, psychological, and spiritual needs • choosing healthful activities, such as getting enough sleep, spending time with friends, and eating well.	• making a commitment to personal and professional goals through growth and lifelong learning • taking responsibility for one's personal and professional reflective practices, emotional health, and skill development • using proactive and comprehensive strategies for personal and professional growth and development.

Self-stewardship requires that we lead ourselves to make informed decisions, take initiative, and advocate for sufficient resources to achieve our goals. We do this work of self-stewardship because no one else can. When we make determinations about what we are accountable for in our work, we can then plan and advocate for our well-being. Part of the work of self-stewardship involves honestly identifying our strengths and limitations that allow us to know when we can achieve something on our own and when we need support. Each of us comes to this work with internal and external resources. Internal resources can include aspects of our personalities, such as our motivations, drives, and approaches for engaging the world. External resources include people or supports, tools, and information from other people—friends, colleagues, family members, or the larger community. We can be a good steward as we access and use these resources to manage our well-being in our personal and professional lives.

Self-stewardship starts with self-leadership. We practice self-leadership when we engage in the following:

- **Self-awareness**: understanding our abilities, limitations, values, beliefs, and emotions.

- **Self-motivation**: working toward meaningful, achievable goals; sustaining motivation and resolving challenges.

- **Self-regulation**: managing our emotions and behaviors through the self-discipline of our personal and professional practices.

- **Self-confidence**: trusting ourselves and our decision-making as well as valuing our unique skills and characteristics.

- **Self-accountability**: taking responsibility for ourselves and our actions and honoring commitments.

Identifying Self-Stewardship Actions

In this activity, use the self-leadership concepts to reflect on your personal and professional practices.

	IN MY PERSONAL LIFE	IN MY PROFESSIONAL LIFE
Self-Awareness What are my abilities, limitations, values, beliefs, and emotions?		
Self-Motivation How do I stay motivated as I work toward meaningful goals?		
Self-Regulation How do I manage my emotions and behaviors?		
Self-Confidence How do I trust myself and my decision-making, recognizing my unique skills and characteristics?		
Self-Accountability How do I take responsibility for myself and my actions and honor my commitments?		

Reflecting on our own self-leadership practices supports us in managing our lives. Self-stewardship is both care for ourselves and an awareness of how our choices impact those around us. It provides a foundation for sustaining proactive, intentional, and holistic approaches to well-being that support our continuous personal and professional growth.

Self-Stewardship in Practice

To focus and sustain our physical, emotional, cognitive, social, psychological, and spiritual health, we must take intentional actions and make conscious decisions. We must identify our personal and professional needs, establish limits, and partake in routines and activities that enhance our general well-being. Self-stewardship includes a range of habits and behaviors that promote personal development, decision-making, and goal setting related to our well-being. Choosing to change habits can be hard work. In changing habits, we are building new pathways in the brain to change our behaviors. Also, remember to engage in self-compassion as a practice of well-being as you work towards change because there are times when you will struggle as well as succeed.

Actions that help us build and sustain our changing habits include developing new personal and professional skills, practicing self-reflection, and appraising our emotions. Activities for self-stewardship involve setting goals, prioritizing self-care, seeking feedback, managing our time, pursuing reflective practices, and building professional skills.

ACTIVITY 4.2

Making Changes and Practicing Them

→ What is one area in which you believe you could be a better steward?

→ → What would you need to change in your practices or habits? (Name a few.)

→ → → How could you motivate yourself to maintain those changes?

→ → → → How would you know you've succeeded over time?

The Need for Boundaries in Our Work

Self-stewardship is a type of self-leadership that embraces looking inward and accepts that taking care of ourselves is our own responsibility. In this practice, we acknowledge that when we rely on others to tell us what we can and cannot do—or ask others to be responsible for our work-life balance—we are engaging in unhealthy behaviors. Centering our work in ethical practices supports us in defining our **professional boundaries**. Our **professional identities** influence the boundaries we set around work.

Individuals in helping professions often struggle with personal and professional boundaries (Osgood 2012). The personal and professional selves can become entangled in early childhood practices when we mix "who we are" with "what we do." Consider the last time you gave up something you needed in service to your work—for example, staying late to provide extra attention or support for a child or family when you needed to leave on time for rest and recovery. Decisions about when to care for yourself and when to care for others can be complex in the early childhood education profession because of the collaborative nature of the work that hinges on and exists for relationships with others. As a profession, we work for agreement and discourage challenges with the children and families we serve. Knowing that early childhood has highly permeable boundaries because of the emotional nature of the work reminds us that we need to be extra vigilant in developing and maintaining boundaries.

People who work in helping professions and who have a professional identity that involves caring for others are motivated to uphold the well-being of others and maintain positive relationships. While admirable, this approach to work can lead to poorly clarified professional boundaries and result in unhealthy altruistic or self-sacrificing practices. We often think about our work and spend emotional energy on our profession long after our workdays are over. Research shows that **altruism** (or selflessness) is a common trait in early childhood educators, who often sacrifice their own personal well-being for the children in their classrooms or communities (Taggart 2019). Related research explores how a need to be "good"—as in the "good early childhood educator"—often affects individuals who identify as female more than those who identify as male (Langford 2006). Connecting one's worth to—or defining it by—being "good" leads to extreme altruism, which creates habits of self-sacrifice that increase burnout in the helping professions.

Analyzing Altruistic Behaviors

Professional sustainability means reflecting on your actions and analyzing the beliefs behind any altruistic behaviors. Reflect on the following statements and rate yourself on the scale.

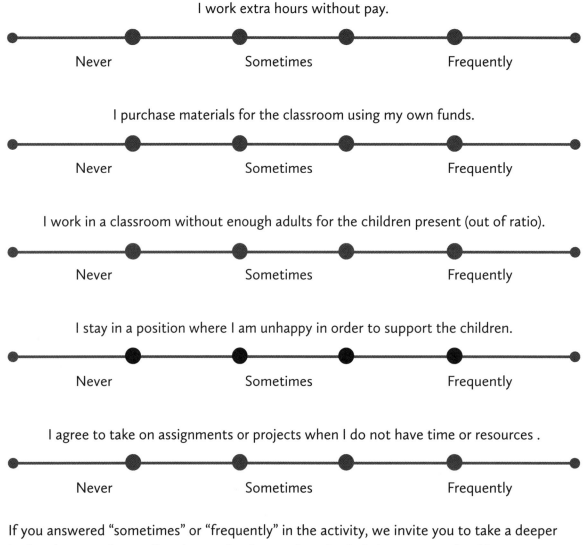

I work extra hours without pay.

Never — Sometimes — Frequently

I purchase materials for the classroom using my own funds.

Never — Sometimes — Frequently

I work in a classroom without enough adults for the children present (out of ratio).

Never — Sometimes — Frequently

I stay in a position where I am unhappy in order to support the children.

Never — Sometimes — Frequently

I agree to take on assignments or projects when I do not have time or resources .

Never — Sometimes — Frequently

If you answered "sometimes" or "frequently" in the activity, we invite you to take a deeper look at how you internalize the need to be good or altruistic in your practice. You may be engaging in self-sacrificing behaviors that are created by poorly clarified professional boundaries.

This exercise may have made you uncomfortable or brought up strong emotions. If so, this could mean you have internalized the message that self-sacrifice and altruistic behaviors are necessary in being a "good early childhood educator." Building professional boundaries using the tools available to our profession will support you to do the important work of self-stewardship.

Using the Code of Ethical Conduct to Build Better Boundaries

For educators who are struggling to determine professional boundaries, the **NAEYC Code of Ethical Conduct** is an invaluable resource. First, the code outlines the core responsibilities of early childhood educators. These include responsibilities to children and families, colleagues and programs, and the larger society. The code goes further in helping us determine where professional responsibilities begin and end. As you encounter a challenge, use the code to help you decide if something is a professional responsibility or not. We will explore the Code of Ethical Conduct in greater depth in chapter 6.

https://www
.naeyc.org
/resources
/position
-statements
/ethical-conduct

Second, when thinking about professional boundaries, the messages we tell ourselves and others are critically important. If, in the previous exercise, you discovered that you were tempted to equate altruistic behaviors with being a good educator, then thinking about this internal messaging might be helpful. Consider the table below that provides new scripts to defend boundaries and replace overly altruistic internal messages. Practicing this kind of messaging will increase your skills in self-stewardship.

POORLY CLARIFIED PROFESSIONAL BOUNDARIES: ALTRUISTIC MESSAGING	CLARIFIED STRONG PROFESSIONAL BOUNDARIES: SELF-STEWARDSHIP MESSAGING
I can work extra hours without pay.	Professionals are paid for their work. Work includes both teaching and preparation time.
I use my own funds for materials for the classroom.	Programs need to resource their classrooms. It is the program's responsibility to ensure that all basic materials are in good working order.
When needed, I work out of ratio.	Professionals are not asked by their programs to violate state laws or the NAEYC Code of Ethical Conduct.
I stay for the children.	Ethical responsibilities include care for self. Emotionally healthy early childhood educators support emotionally healthy classrooms.
I agree to do projects even when under-resourced.	I take time to reflect about my interest level and resources before making a decision to take on a new project.

Building Strong Professional Boundaries

Building strong professional boundaries means establishing healthy professional practices. These practices have their foundation in the skills we covered earlier:

- **Self-awareness** supports strong boundaries through an awareness of your own needs, values, and limits. It helps you recognize when a **boundary** has been crossed, protecting your well-being.
- **Self-motivation** determines your self-advocacy, how you follow through in setting and maintaining boundaries when prioritizing well-being.
- **Self-regulation** includes managing your emotions, actions, and behaviors in ways that are consistent with your boundaries. It involves responding, rather than reacting, when your boundaries are tested.
- **Self-confidence** centers on knowing your own value to confidently express your demands, limitations, and boundaries without feeling fear or guilt when others challenge or criticize them.
- **Self-accountability** embraces reflecting on your boundaries so you adjust them as needed. It includes being cognitive of and consistent in enforcing your boundaries.

ACTIVITY 4.4

Clarifying Boundaries

While it can be difficult, examining your boundaries is some of the most important work you will do to practice self-stewardship. When your boundaries remain flexible, you will take on more than you have the resources to handle, leading to fatigue and burnout. Below, reflect on your answers in activity 4.3, or choose some boundaries that you know are challenging for you at work. Next, think about how you can make changes in your professional practices to strengthen your professional boundaries.

FLEXIBLE PROFESSIONAL BOUNDARIES	CHANGES IN PRACTICES TO STRENGTHEN BOUNDARIES

Proactively engaging in self-stewardship involves accessing resources and establishing and upholding boundaries to support emotional health and well-being. Self-stewardship presents exciting opportunities not only for advancing individual well-being but also for changing the culture of the profession. Individuals who are good stewards and ensure their individual well-being will promote a profession that values strong professional boundaries.

Reflection on Practice

Let's review the questions from the beginning of the chapter.

What is self-stewardship?

How do we practice self-stewardship?

Why center ethics and boundaries in our work?

How do we build strong professional boundaries?

CHAPTER 5

Barriers to Self-Stewardship

Demands are requests on one's physical, emotional, cognitive, social, psychological, or spiritual resources that require energy to address.

S elf-stewardship requires us to make choices that support our health, happiness, and well-being and use our resources wisely. To make choices that are physically, emotionally, cognitively, socially, psychologically, and spiritually sustaining, we need to recognize demands and **barriers**. *Demands* are requests on our resources, and they require energy to address. *Barriers* are obstacles that can keep us from successfully managing demands. Recognizing demands and the barriers we face in meeting them is a critical component of removing the obstacles that prevent us from meeting our goals. In this chapter, we ask the following questions:

- What are demands?
- What are our perceptions of demands?
- What are the barriers impacting our self-stewardship?
- How do we navigate systemic barriers?

Identifying Demands

Every day, we navigate expectations, tasks, and responsibilities that researchers of stress and coping identify as *demands.* Demands are requests or requirements on our time, energy, attention, skills, and so on. It may seem harsh to talk about things like work hours and car-pools as *demands*, but these are requirements in our lives that take resources. In more common language, we might refer to these as *stressors*, but there is a subtle difference between demands and stressors. Demands are more global and routine, and they do not always cause stress. They are simply requests on our resources.

Demands can come from external and internal sources. For example, your job may require that you report to work from seven o'clock in the morning until three o'clock in the afternoon, but also asks that you be available in the evenings to respond to parent emails. These are examples of external sources of demands. Some examples of internal demands include your unique needs for caring for your physical health, such as rest and exercise, as well as other requirements you place on yourself related to your own motivations and values, such as being creative in your work or feeling socially present. Well-being is influenced by both internal and external demands.

Demands, both internal and external, are often competing, such as wanting to spend time with family yet needing to balance work and home. For example, the demand to be at work at seven o'clock in the morning can compete with the need to drop off your child at school and speak to their teacher at seven thirty. In this example, external demands (time requirements, the need to be in two places) and internal demands (values associated with being a trustworthy worker and a present parent) are in play. Internally competing demands can cause stress in our lives, such as when we make choices that involve our values or beliefs or that affect our sociocultural, personal, or professional identities.

Stress occurs when we perceive that we are being asked to do something (demands) larger than we can manage with our toolboxes (resources). When we feel that we have the resources we need, we can cope with the small and large demands in our lives. However, without the resources we need, stressors add up over time and damage our health and well-being.

Our Perceptions of Demands

It is important to remember that it is our *perception*, or what we think about the demands and resources, that affects our stress levels. The work of appraising the demands and resources in our professional work can be difficult, but it is a necessary part of understanding potential sources of stress. When we reflect on the demands that are placed on us as part of our work, and the resources we have to address the demands, we might find that some of the demands are easily met with the resources we have, and others are not. We also might discover that some of the demands we think are external are actually more related to internal values. Not all demands are problematic. Meeting demands makes life and work interesting, motivating, and fulfilling. However, when we don't feel that we have the ability to meet the demands, we can experience stress. When all the requests in life seem overwhelming, consider the following questions:

- What is the current demand I am perceiving, and what is the source? Is this demand internal or external?
- Do I feel I have the resources to meet the demand?
- Is there a conflict between this demand and others? Does using resources for this demand mean I don't have resources to meet another?

In this next activity, we are going to take a close look at some demands that early childhood educators might experience. When you read the statements, consider whether the demand is internal or external and whether it is easily met or a challenge to meet with existing resources.

Thinking about Demands

Looking at this list of demands, circle whether you see the demand as internal or external and as easily met or challenging.

I have to make sure that children have all of the materials necessary for learning, even if I have to purchase them myself.

Internal or External   Easily Met or Challenging

I am responsible for supporting all of the children in my classroom, regardless of their behavior or challenges. For example, I must support a child who bit another child.

Internal or External   Easily Met or Challenging

I am responsible for keeping the classroom clean and should clean the table after snack.

Internal or External   Easily Met or Challenging

It is my responsibility to make sure that all teachers are doing their best for the children. When a member of the team is late, I have to have a conversation with my coworker.

Internal or External   Easily Met or Challenging

I am responsible for keeping children safe at all times, so I must watch the children on the playground even though it is my break time.

Internal or External   Easily Met or Challenging

Add your own statement.

Internal or External   Easily Met or Challenging

Reflect on your answers to the questions above. What did you notice about the sources of these demands and your feelings about the resources you have to meet them? While there are likely many internal and external demands that are easily met, those we find challenging—whether from within ourselves or from our contexts—can alert us to the need for self-stewardship work. A difficulty in meeting demands can signal the presence of a barrier. In the next section, we turn our attention to what keeps us from being able to easily meet demands and practice self-stewardship.

Barriers to Self-Stewardship

Barriers exist all around us, keeping us from certain pathways and spaces. Not all barriers are bad; some can keep us from harm. However, barriers that keep us from self-stewardship need a critical look. As we begin to unpack the barriers to self-stewardship, it can be helpful to set aside the temptation to think about how we might "overcome" or "respond" or "defeat" the barrier. Instead, we invite you to take a moment to pause and just notice those things that keep you from engaging in self-stewardship. We are going to look at the fences or the mountains and not make plans to climb them.

A barrier is "a fence or other obstacle that prevents movement or access" (Oxford University Press 2018). These fences or obstacles keep us from well-being. External barriers exist outside of us and act as a fence, keeping us from the greener pasture of self-stewardship. **External barriers** can include environmental factors such as culture, policies, finances, or discrimination, or a lack of emotional support or professional skills. For example, low wages in the early childhood profession can create financial difficulties that lead to barriers in accessing housing and health care, which in turn affect how someone manages stress and maintains well-being. **Internal barriers** are within ourselves and can include negative thinking patterns or emotional reactions, as well as self-doubt and unhealthy habits. Without adequate and effective coping skills, addressing the negative thinking patterns that create a sense of isolation and keep us from seeking emotional support from others can be a struggle.

These are some barriers commonly identified in the early childhood profession:

- too much work required
- policies that promote unhealthy practices, placing more than typical stress on educators working directly with children
- a program culture that does not support self-stewardship
- a program culture that allows bias and discrimination against self-stewardship choices
- work that promotes negative emotions
- work that promotes unhealthy habits

The barriers we experience in these systems are not all the same. Just like demands, barriers come from our contexts (external sources) and also from within ourselves (internal sources). As we think about internal and external barriers, some are within our control, and others are not. Noticing the barriers is a first step, but we also need to recognize the difference between barriers in our personal self-stewardship and in our professional self-stewardship. As we shared in chapter 1, the parts of self are intertwined. Personal barriers to self-stewardship impact our professional selves and vice versa. As we continue to think carefully about barriers, let's consider this connection.

Identifying External and Internal Barriers

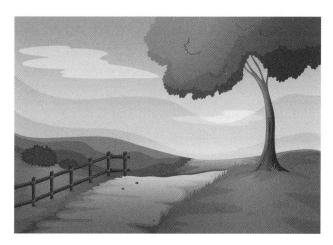

Make an **external barriers** visual. For example, you might draw a road leading to a self-stewardship destination. Now add to your drawing any barriers that are keeping you from your self-stewardship practice. Focus on those things *outside* of yourself that keep you from reaching self-stewardship and wellness. External barriers are often easy to identify but hard to address.

Return to your drawing and think about **internal barriers** you carry that keep you from self-stewardship. Some common examples are guilt and feeling unworthy. You might want to draw these differently from the external barriers, perhaps as things you carry like baggage. Make as complete a list as possible.

Ask yourself these questions as you reflect on your visual:

- What do you notice about the drawing?
- Does it seem to capture everything?

Navigating Systemic Barriers

Internal and external barriers are all reinforced by the characteristics of our environments. As we work to notice the sources of barriers, it is important to acknowledge that larger systems play a role in supporting and upholding them. These systems have characteristics that help or hinder self-stewardship efforts. An example of a barrier might be how program supervision is viewed. Visits from a supervisor can be seen as supporting or critiquing classroom practices. If the visit is seen as a partnership to improve practices, then the system (program) is open to an exchange of ideas and problem solving. If we identify the supervisor as a critic of our skills and practices, then we might close ourselves off from the feedback. Our self-stewardship is affected by our interpretation of the supervisor's visit to our classroom.

While a complete review of systems theory is beyond the scope of this book, it is important to understand a little about the types of systems as we think more deeply about barriers. At the most simplistic level, systems can be characterized as open or closed. *Open systems* welcome external influences and good communication, while *closed systems* isolate those inside, with rigid lines and secret keeping. These concepts can be applied to early childhood programs and other systems in the profession, and can help us understand how systems support or inhibit practices of self-stewardship.

Early childhood programs that are **open systems** have open boundaries that create transparency among members of the early childhood community—educators, families, and children. These systems invite families into classroom communities. They have responsive and shared decision-making practices and a shared understanding of how and why educators work with young children. They welcome new ideas and practices. Decisions in open systems uphold ethical practices.

Closed systems are isolated and self-contained. Closed early childhood systems may be under-resourced or feature an uneven distribution of resources. Their decision-making processes are unclear and may be arbitrary. In these systems, individuals work in isolation, and each educator's plans, including their motivations or reasons for teaching, are separate and often adjacent to the actual practices in the classrooms, programs, or schools. Closed systems minimize outside contact and are resistant to change, reinforcing messages that historic practices are best.

Reflecting on Open and Closed Systems

Writing and drawing on the circles below, reflect on open and closed early childhood systems. What are the characteristics (rules, beliefs, and actions) of open and closed early childhood systems?

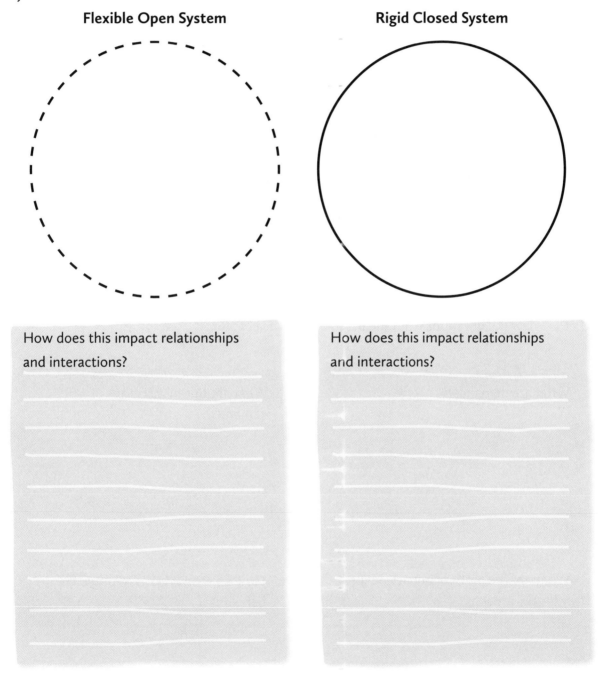

Flexible Open System

Rigid Closed System

How does this impact relationships and interactions?

How does this impact relationships and interactions?

So how do systems relate to barriers? Barriers within systems, especially those that restrict movement and access to information, are frequently put in place to benefit people in power. For example, many state initiatives are calling for bachelor's degrees in early childhood education without providing scholarships or additional pay upon graduating. States making these decisions without understanding the challenges early childhood educators face when obtaining additional degrees is an example of a closed system making decisions without considering educators' experiences. These growing pains of our profession demonstrate that systemic and individual needs are not yet aligned, leading to unrealistic pressures on early childhood educators. This type of pressure affects well-being when the tension between a system and an individual puts all of the expectations on the individual to meet the system demands.

The idea that a system or profession could have an impact in the unwellness of employees is a difficult and uncomfortable recognition. But remember—we are just noticing. We are not placing blame, and we are not yet talking about how we can overcome it. Instead, we are taking time to lead ourselves through the work and make decisions to support our own well-being. In coming sections, we will get to proactive actions to influence the profession. For now, let's keep the focus on ourselves, noticing how these complex and critical questions directly and indirectly impact our ability to practice self-stewardship.

Reflecton on Practice

Let's review the questions from the beginning of the chapter

What are demands?	What are our perceptions of demands?

What are the barriers impacting our self-stewardship?	How do we navigate systemic barriers?

PART 3

Professional Skills: Filling Our Toolboxes

In the first two sections of the workbook, we reflected on well-being and explored self-stewardship as emotionally meaningful and fulfilling work.

Self-stewardship is the ability to lead one's physical, emotional, cognitive, social, psychological, and spiritual self in ways that actively promote and sustain one's well-being. It involves self-awareness, self-motivation, self-regulation, self-confidence, self-accountability, and professional boundaries. One of the challenges of self-stewardship is navigating demands. Stress occurs when we feel we can't meet the demands placed on us. Further, barriers can make it difficult for us to meet the demands we experience in systems, and systems reinforce the barriers. Engaging in the process of *noticing* allows us to think first about the sources of the demands and barriers that keep us from our wellness work.

While we likely cannot quickly change the demands, barriers, and systems we experience in our work, we can make decisions about how we engage in professional practices. We should work for change in our systems and to overcome barriers but we can only engage in this work when we start from a place of well-being. In part 3, we explore some of the tools in our profession that can help us with this work as we engage in our professional practices. We look to fill our toolboxes with skills to navigate the big and small challenges we face every day. Chapters 6 through 8 address the barriers and demands we face in our work and help us identify resources in our professional practices. Chapters 9 and 10 focus on problem-solving using the skills from our toolbox.

Self-stewardship requires that we focus on our professional identity when making informed decisions in our practices. We start in chapter 6 by strengthening our professional identities. Self-stewardship further requires that we have—or can identify and access—sufficient resources to reach and achieve our goals. Acknowledging our strengths and limitations and seeking supports are part of filling our toolboxes. Chapter 7 focuses on identifying and accessing resources for our emotional work. Chapter 8 builds our interpersonal skills in a professional setting. Chapter 9 looks at how to make choices that support well-being as we solve problems every day. Chapter 10 highlights how to appraise these everyday choices with the skills from this workbook, using the Problem-Solving Pathway.

Much of our well-being is guided by our self-stewardship in daily choices. Think back to activity 3.3, where we conducted a first appraisal of our coping skills and the resources we might need. We come back to the work here by identifying resources to support self-stewardship and well-being. Consider this scenario:

Molly's mother drops her off during the morning gathering. You are working with your coteacher to bring a group of excited children together. Molly's mother leans over and shares, "I need to talk with you now." Your emotions are torn: if you leave your coteacher, she will struggle to start the morning gathering. On the other hand, you want to make sure you address Molly's mother's concerns. What do you do?

Scenarios like the one above are common in early childhood programs, where we can face many competing priorities. Having a professional identity grounded in the NAEYC Code of Ethical Conduct clarifies our responsibilities to children, families, and colleagues and serves as the starting point for all reflections on professional practices. But what skills and tools would we need to make decisions and solve this problem?

If this scenario were shared in a professional development workshop or training, the first responses might involve **professional skills**. For example: How do you talk with the parents? What are classroom management strategies that create space for children's autonomy when you need to speak to an adult? However, perpetually responding to crises without self-stewardship is unsustainable. To employ self-stewardship, we center reflective practices, identifying and accessing emotional support to create a model for well-being.

To center **reflective practices**, we ask questions such as these: How might you reflect on the emotions of the experience? How can you create a mental model to help you in the future? Engaging in reflection creates opportunities to look at our practices in new ways. Reflection can also be helpful for recognizing the emotional work involved in an experience.

The **emotional support** needed to do this work, or even a recognition of the emotions involved, is frequently absent. Developing a strong relationship with families is emotional work. Some relationships are full of joy, and others are strained and difficult. The scenario does not give us any insight into the status of the relationship between the teacher and Molly's mom, whether it is a good relationship with trust and respect or one that is strained and challenging. What we know is that the teacher likely experiences emotions in conjunction with such an event, including worry, anxiety, anger, resentment, frustration, concern, fatigue, and so on. In this scenario, we can see how the demands of Molly's family need to be met with reflective practices, emotional work, and professional skills. No skills exist in isolation. Instead, solutions come from across skill sets and are grounded in knowing who we are as educators.

CHAPTER 6

Building a Strong Professional Identity

Our professional identity is our attitudes, values, knowledge, beliefs, and skills, framed by our Code of Ethics and enacted at the individual level in our professional practice.

As we build the professional practices that will support self-stewardship, we need to start with a clear understanding of our professional identity. Each of us has a professional identity that differentiates between our personal and professional self. Our professional identity follows our professional code of conduct. We attend to our well-being by practicing skills that sustain our professional identity. In early childhood education, our work is guided by the NAEYC Code of Ethical Conduct. As early childhood education is a diverse profession, you may also follow codes of conduct for overlapping professions, such as for home visiting or infant mental health. In this chapter, we ask the following:

- What is a professional identity?
- What are the barriers to developing a professional identity?
- How are our professional identities connected to professional values, ethics, and practices?
- What helps us promote professional well-being?

Our Professional Identity

Our professional identity is built from a set of core values and beliefs as agreed on by a professional community. In early childhood education, our values and beliefs are outlined in NAEYC's Code of Ethical Conduct. Our professional identity emerges as we internalize our profession's core values and beliefs.

- Who am I in the lives of young children?
- What is important to me in my work?
- How do I define professionalism?
- How does my work contribute to my sense of self and my well-being?

The early childhood structures in which we work and the ways we are prepared through education and professional development affect how we form our professional identity. These structures and methods of preparation vary widely in the early childhood profession.

Barriers to a Strong Professional Identity

Developing a strong professional early childhood identity can be difficult, as educators face many external and internal pressures as outlined in chapter 5. Some external impacts on professional identity formation (that is, what keeps you from being recognized as a professional) are the lack or uneven presentation of the following:

- public recognition of early childhood as a profession
- fair wages
- professional preparation
- understanding of the uniqueness of childhood as distinct time in life

Internal factors on professional identity formation include:

- energy to sustain productivity and handle workload
- desire for choice and control (autonomy)
- sense of belonging
- sense of purpose, the worthiness of the work

So how do we overcome these barriers? What can we do about these structural problems in our profession? We begin by building a strong professional identity and clarifying our own commitment to our professional responsibilities. We look to the Code of Ethical Conduct as the foundation of our work. If we consider our professional identity as a garden, then we can visualize how to cultivate ourselves, just as we care for a garden. Nutrient-rich environments include the resources of time, mentorship, and community. If one of the three is missing in our practice or organizations, then we do not have all the nutrients that we need to thrive.

Professional Values, Ethics, and Practice

The NAEYC Code of Ethical Conduct is a powerful tool for creating a professional identity and for facing our challenges because it provides a framework for decision-making and problem solving. Educators can use the code to guide their practice, support ongoing professional development, promote ethical leadership, and advocate for themselves as well as children, families, and the profession.

When we are faced with difficult decisions, the Code of Ethical Conduct helps us choose ethically. When we make our professional decisions based on the code, we operate within a framework of professional practices and exhibit the characteristic of **professionalism**. Professionalism is based on a shared set of professional values that guide the actions of a profession and its practice, not any one person's values, attitudes, and beliefs.

NAEYC Code of Ethical Conduct

- Code of Ethical Conduct and Statement of Commitment (English and Spanish)
- Supplement for Early Childhood Program Administrators
- Supplement for Early Childhood Adult Educators

There are two main books to learn more about the Code of Ethical Conduct:

- *Ethics and the Early Childhood Educator*, second edition
- *Teaching the NAEYC Code of Ethical Conduct: A Resource Guide*, revised edition

https://www
.naeyc.org
/resources
/position
-statements
/ethical-conduct

The first and most important principle in our profession is this:

> *Principle P-1.1—Above all, we shall not harm children. We shall not participate in practices that are emotionally damaging, physically harmful, disrespectful, degrading, dangerous, exploitative, or intimidating to children. This principle has precedence over all others in this Code.* (NAEYC 2011, 4)

With this grounding, the Code of Ethical Conduct goes on to outline our four core responsibilities to children, families, colleagues, and the larger society. These professional responsibilities are the foundation for the development of our professional identity, including professional attitudes, values, knowledge, beliefs, and skills. In this next activity, we start with these four responsibilities and spend some time building our own statements about how they inform our professional identity. These statements may be useful as you share your work and philosophies with others, both within and outside of the profession.

Professional Values and the Code of Ethics

In this activity, reflect on your own practice using the core responsibilities outlined in the NAEYC Code of Ethical Conduct (see QR code on previous page). As you review the code, consider what it says about each responsibility, then finish the statement in your own words, connecting it to your professional identity by completing the sentences "I am a teacher who" and "This guides my practice by."

ETHICAL RESPONSIBILITY	WHAT IT SAYS IN THE CODE OF ETHICAL CONDUCT IN YOUR OWN WORDS	PROFESSIONAL IDENTITY STATEMENT I AM A TEACHER WHO . . .	THIS GUIDES MY PRACTICE BY . . .
Children			
Families			
Colleagues			
Community and society			

When we refer to the code to make daily decisions about our practices, it informs our individual professional conduct. When multiple teachers or administrators in a program and across programs do this work individually, the code can promote a culture of ethical practice and leadership. The code also informs advocacy efforts, including the development of policies, routines, and systems that focus on sustainable practices to protect the core responsibilities. Finally, the code informs professional development decisions, including how and when we engage in reflective practice. Understanding our professional identity can give us a window into our professional wellness.

Promoting Professional Wellness

So how does our professional identity inform or help us with professional wellness? Understanding our professional identity can take us only so far because we do not exist only as professional beings; our professional identities are informed and reinforced by our personal identities. Personal identities are rooted in our values and beliefs, or what we believe to be right, true, and good. For early childhood educators, this connection is frequently experienced as the personal "why" behind the professional work. This might be a personal story about how a teacher impacted their life, a lesson that they believe is critically important for young children, or a commitment to social justice in which the education and care of young children is a critical component. The "why" is as varied and diverse as the individual early childhood teachers. We all have a story of how we came to work in early childhood. Part of the development of a holistic professional self is nurturing a strong connection to our personal "why" or our purpose for doing the work. We acknowledge that our personal and professional selves are intertwined. Most early childhood teachers do this work for deeply personal reasons.

In this next activity, we invite you to reflect on the NAEYC Statement of Commitment and connect it to your personal "why."

ACTIVITY 6.2

Translating the Statement of Commitment

To connect the NAEYC Statement of Commitment (NAEYC 2011, 9) to your personal "why," read the individual statement and then record what comes to mind. It might be a story from your own life or teaching experience, or it might be connected to a personal value. Then in the final column, record your response to the statement: "I am committed to this because . . ."

STATEMENT	PERSONAL CONNECTIONS	I AM COMMITTED TO THIS BECAUSE . . .
"Never harm children."		
"Ensure that programs for young children are based on current knowledge and research of child development and early childhood education."		

STATEMENT	PERSONAL CONNECTIONS	I AM COMMITTED TO THIS BECAUSE . . .
"Respect and support families in their task of nurturing children."		
"Respect colleagues in early childhood care and education and support them in maintaining the NAEYC Code of Ethical Conduct."		
"Serve as an advocate for children, their families, and their teachers in community and society. Stay informed of and maintain high standards of professional conduct."		
"Engage in an ongoing process of self-reflection, realizing that personal characteristics, biases, and beliefs have an impact on children and families."		
"Be open to new ideas and be willing to learn from the suggestions of others."		
"Continue to learn, grow, and contribute as a professional."		
"Honor the ideals and principles of the NAEYC Code of Ethical Conduct."		

A strong professional identity that is framed by a strong personal identity, including your personal story, can help sustain the work, even in the face of challenges. So how do we know if our practices are working? In the final section of this chapter, we turn to methods for reflecting on our professional well-being.

Reflecting on Professional Well-Being

A strong professional identity informs professional practices and self-stewardship. Creating and maintaining this connection and balance between your professional and personal lives supports you in not sacrificing one for the other. Professional self-stewardship includes developing the professional, reflective, and emotional skills needed to succeed in early childhood. The following activity is an opportunity to refocus on well-being as a holistic, professional, and essential practice. Use this tool to reflect on (1) what is present, (2) what you want more of in your personal and professional self, and (3) what professional actions you would like to try next.

ACTIVITY 6.3

The Professional Wellness Wheel

Circle the answers that are correct for you most of the time. Feel free to add other questions that might be specific to you and your professional context.

Physical Wellness

Y	N	I am generally free from illness.
Y	N	I have the stamina needed to do my work.
Y	N	I take lunch breaks.
Y	N	I take time off when sick.
Y	N	Other: _____

Emotional Wellness

Y	N	I assume that everyone acts with positive intention.
Y	N	I can communicate my needs in my professional life.
Y	N	I make emotionally healthy decisions for myself and my classroom.
Y	N	I seek help from others when I need support (skills or emotional support).
Y	N	Other: _____

Cognitive Wellness

Y	N	I read professional magazines and journals.
Y	N	I commit time and focus to professional self-development.
Y	N	I engage in professional development in a variety of settings (in person or online).
Y	N	I subscribe to and follow a professional code of ethics in my decision-making.
Y	N	Other: _____

Social Wellness

Y	N	I reflect on my practices or consult with a more experienced colleague.
Y	N	I have a sense of belonging and not isolation in my work.
Y	N	I can resolve conflicts in the workplace.
Y	N	I have clear boundaries between myself and families or clients.
Y	N	Other: _____

Psychological Wellness

Y	N	I keep a notebook or journal on my professional practices.
Y	N	I do not engage in gossip.
Y	N	I do not answer email, texts, or calls outside of work hours.
Y	N	I keep my personal and professional social media separate.
Y	N	Other: _____

Spiritual Wellness

Y	N	I find meaning and purpose in my work.
Y	N	I understand my professional values, attitudes, and beliefs.
Y	N	I am a part of a group where I can trust others and expect trust in return
Y	N	I communicate about what is important to me and do not compromise my professional values.
Y	N	Other: _____

For each of the questions to which you answered yes, fill in one segment on the wheel in the corresponding category. Now take a few minutes to fill in the wheel. For each yes, fill in a section of the correct segment on the wheel.

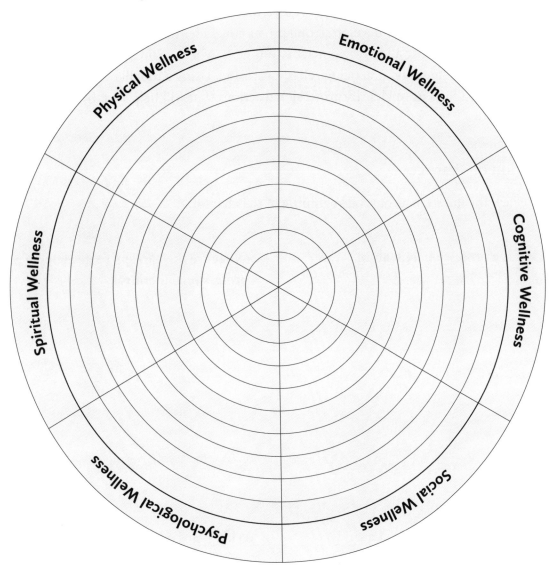

Step back and look at the completed wheel. What areas do you notice as being especially strong? Are there areas you are missing? As you reflect on your professional wellness in the activity, you may have discovered that you are experiencing a great deal of wellness in some areas of your life but less in other areas. Since each of these domains contributes to our overall professional well-being, it is important to remember and give room for every area. If you are looking for ways to increase your well-being in a domain, go back and look at the statements for ideas. Be careful about jumping to an action plan or adding to your to-do list. Remember to treat yourself compassionately as you notice areas for growth or opportunity.

Building a strong professional identity can guide and protect our professional practices. The NAEYC Code of Ethical Conduct provides a road map to support our professional practices and decisions as we develop strong professional identities. We can keep our professional identities strong and bring impact to our work when we integrate a personal "why" while pursuing wellness and practicing self-stewardship. Using a tool like a professional wellness wheel allows us to identify professional actions that will help sustain our professional identities.

Reflection on Practice

Let's review the questions from the beginning of the chapter.

What is a professional identity?

What are the barriers to developing a professional identity?

How are our professional identities connected to professional values, ethics, and practices?

What helps us promote professional well-being?

CHAPTER 7

Identifying and Accessing Emotional Support

Emotional well-being is the quality of emotional responses to life experiences, including the ability to adapt and change, demonstrate resiliency, resolve conflicts, manage emotions, and generate consistent feelings of happiness and hopefulness.

I n this chapter, we will dig deep to identify practices that help us reinforce our emotional well-being. We start by noticing that emotional well-being does not occur in isolation. Rather, our work exists in a framework of overlapping environments, each with its own emotional context. Within these spaces, our relationships provide us with connection, support, purpose, and improved mental and physical health, all of which are essential for emotional well-being. In this chapter, we ask the following questions:

- What do we need to know to navigate our emotional work?
- How do our emotional connections build our social support systems?
- How do we identify our support system resources?
- How do we build our social supports?

Navigating Our Emotional Work

To identify and engage in emotional work, we need a basic understanding of emotions and how they function in our everyday lives. Emotions are a natural part of the human experience and are neither good nor bad. Our emotions are revealed through both unconscious actions (think of body language or facial expressions) and conscious actions (think of how we express ourselves to others). Our emotions are part of our communication tools, which we use to signal our senses of belonging, love, and connection, as well as our frustration, hurt, or distress, among many other emotions. Emotions are transmissible, and we can influence others' emotions both positively and negatively. Because of this, we need to be able to regulate our emotions to build and sustain healthy relationships.

Our emotions are highly individualized, connecting to our experiences and culture, ranging from simple to complex. A simple subjective emotional experience might be your reaction to seeing a color; a complex one might encompass your competing emotions about your profession. Each person's history creates a different response: one early childhood educator may view the first day with a new class as exciting and challenging, and another teacher may see the work as overwhelming and difficult. Subjective experiences are layered in many emotions, and those emotions tangle together to create our complex emotional lives.

Across cultures, at least six **universal emotions** (sometimes called *basic emotions*)—anger, disgust, fear, happiness, sadness, and surprise—are recognized. Our universal emotions have historic roots in helping us survive. Facial expressions, body language, voice cues, and physiological reactions can all be used to convey these universal emotions. It is also important to note that there are disagreements on the quantity and nature of universal emotions in the field of psychology, and that the categorization of emotions is a complex process that continually evolves over time.

Complex emotions are nuanced adaptations of emotions, which we interpret as we respond to the world around us. They are part of our conscious thought. Emotions overlap, and we often experience many emotions at the same time. While we experience the mind-body sensations of our basic (universal) emotions through the unconscious limbic system, our secondary emotions wind their way more slowly through our **cerebral cortex**, which then supports us in refining our emotions and our responses. This slower process allows us to make conscious choices in how we respond to people and environments.

Our emotions cause complex reactions in our bodies. While many of us can name our emotions and acknowledge their presence in our lives, accepting our emotions is a different skill. When we fail to accept our emotions, we can experience both physical and mental stress. It is not healthy to push our emotions down. Emotional repression works much like pushing a beach ball deep into the water. Think of the energy it takes to hold that beach ball down. Then when we lose control of that beach ball, it shoots to the surface of the water and into the air. The same happens with our emotions: if we push them down, the force of their release is powerful and affects us and those around us. Because our emotions can have far-reaching consequences, especially when not adequately addressed, it is critical that we learn to acknowledge and reflect on our emotions.

Social Support Systems Develop from Our Emotional Connections

Social support systems are the friends, families, colleagues, and communities who support us and encompass the resources we get from other people. These resources help us reflect, handle our emotions, and develop skills. To be emotionally healthy, we need to share our emotions with others, especially when we are emotionally dysregulated. Strong social support systems can amplify our positive emotions too, contributing to our senses of connection and well-being. Without strong social support systems, we lack the safeguards we need to thrive in our lives and work.

We all need social support systems, but few of us access them completely. It is human nature to stand at the bottom of a mountain and think our only choice is to climb alone. Part of the work we do in this workbook is identifying who climbs with us—our social support systems. We are rarely as alone as we think we are. Many of us can name a few key people in our support systems, but we often do not take the time to look at our extended networks. Our social support systems or networks come from not only our circles of family and friends but also our professional colleagues, groups, and organizations that connect with our lives on a regular basis. The common factor is that we know something about the people in these spaces and are, in turn, known by them.

Identifying and building our support systems creates a solid base for our emotional well-being. It is this community that we call on to support our self-stewardship practices. In fact, the act of engaging in self-stewardship often requires a support system. This team influences our thinking and helps us see the opportunities and challenges we face in caring for ourselves. These are the individuals who walk alongside us, cheer us on, or offer resources as we climb. They are not the individuals or organizations who tell us to wait or give up when we expend energy on our journey.

There are different types of social support systems, based on the type of resources we need. Some support systems are focused on decision-making, others help us regulate emotions, and some help us build social connections, also known as *networking*. Some social support systems overlap between our personal and professional lives.

Figure 7.1. Examples of Personal and Professional Social Support Systems

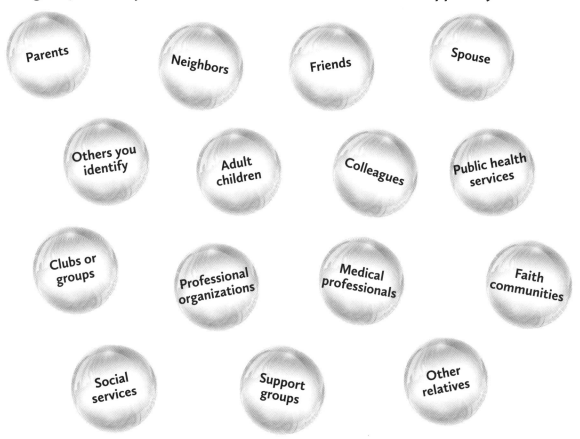

Who else is in your social support system? We can include people in our social support systems when we know them and they are known to us. Who else is in your personal and professional support system?

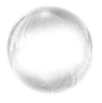 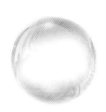 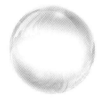 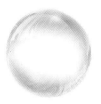

In other words, these are people with whom you can talk about your emotions, people who support your processing and can reflect back on your thinking.

Those of us who work with young children think about support a great deal. We easily recognize that the people in a child's life support their development. A tool to graphically depict these supports is an eco-map. Developed in the 1970s by social worker Ann Hartman, an **eco-map** is a graphic representation (map or drawing) with yourself in the center surrounded by your informal, formal, and intermediate supports. The eco-map is a powerful tool for intentional reflection on support.

ACTIVITY 7.1

Eco-Map of Emotional Supports

The eco-map is inspired by Bronfenbrenner's ecological systems theory (Bronfenbrenner 2005). Your eco-map will be influenced by multiple interacting systems. Create an eco-map for yourself by identifying your supports. A template is provided or you can draw your own eco-map for this activity. Feel free to add to the template, extending your bubbles as needed.

- **Informal supports** go at the top of the eco-map. They consist of family, friends, and neighbors.

- **Formal supports** go at the left of the eco-map. These are professional resources such as a supervisor at work or personal support such as a primary physician.

- **Community supports** go to the right on the eco-map. These are the local organizations you are involved in, such as clubs or spiritual communities.

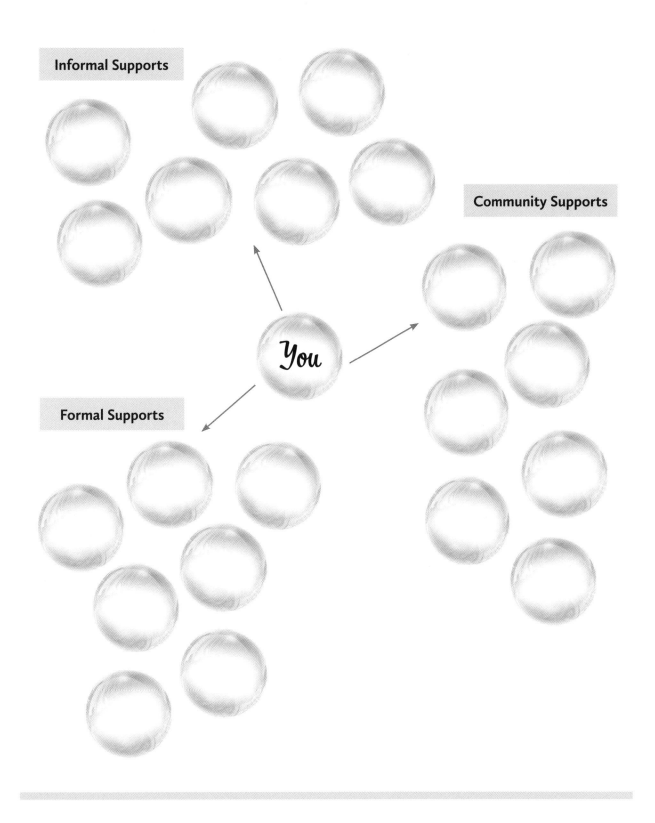

Informal Supports

Community Supports

Formal Supports

You

For the rest of the chapter, we will be revising our eco-maps by examining relationships and supports. Our first appraisal on our eco-map is designed to help us notice our interactions within our social support systems.

Ask yourself these questions and reflect on your answers:

- What do I notice about my support system?
- What emotions do I have when I am with different members of my support system?
- Are there people who create strong positive or negative emotions?
- What might I want to change about whom I engage with?

We can now look more deeply at the emotional health of our relationships at work.

ACTIVITY 7.2

Taking Stock of Relationships in Your Eco-Map

Reflect on each person on your eco-map who connects to your work. Depending on the relationships you have in your work settings, individuals will be in one or more of your informal supports, community supports, or formal supports. Here are some things to attend to:

NAME SOMEONE AT WORK WHO . . .	NAME	THEY DO THIS BY . . .	WHEN I THINK ABOUT THIS INDIVIDUAL, I FEEL . . .	TO MAINTAIN THIS RELATIONSHIP, I HAVE TO . . .
makes you feel inspired.				
makes you feel better.				
makes you feel happy.				

NAME SOMEONE AT WORK WHO . . .	NAME	THEY DO THIS BY . . .	WHEN I THINK ABOUT THIS INDIVIDUAL, I FEEL . . .	TO MAINTAIN THIS RELATIONSHIP, I HAVE TO . . .
makes you feel sad.				
makes you smile.				
makes you feel angry.				
helps you learn.				
acts anxious.				
inspires you to look at your own behavior in new ways.				

Considering who and what in our environment is helping and hurting our work is an important task. Those who are contributing positively are resources. These relationships can be nurtured and fed. Those who are pulling or draining should be managed, or perhaps removed. If you noticed that you could not provide a name for many of the positive prompts, then it is time to proactively seek out support for your network.

Identifying Your Support System's Resources

Each support in one's system offers different social and emotional scaffolding; for example, some are better than others in helping us make decisions, regulate emotions, or build social connections. While there are different ways of classifying social and emotional supports, here are some categories:

- **Instrumental:** support that includes assistance in physical ways. People who give us a ride when our cars don't start, who help us move, or who help us set up an area of the classroom are providing instrumental support. Instrumental support is generally focused on practice or tangible supports in our everyday lives.
- **Informational:** support that involves sharing information, instruction, advice, or ideas. People who help us learn something in our work and people who identify resources for us are providing informational support.
- **Emotional:** support for emotions, including recognition and validation of emotions. People who listen to us and encourage us, who help us laugh, lift our moods, or increase our sense of positivity offer us emotional support.
- **Social:** support that is community-based and organized around a sense of belonging or place. We can find social belonging in a group of individuals or in a larger, more formal organization.

It is not uncommon to have more support in one area over another to experience changes in our systems. When we experience transitions in our lives, our support systems change also, such as when we move or change jobs. It is important to revisit and rebuild support systems after a period of change in our lives or when an area has fewer social or emotional resources.

Some questions you can ask yourself about your support systems include these:

- In looking at my support system, what might be reasons I do not access relatives, friends, or colleagues for support?
- What might be reasons these individuals or groups might not provide support (instrumental, informational, emotional, or social)?
- Are there beliefs, attitudes, or values that prevent the flow of support between us? (Think back to your identified barriers in chapter 5.)

Building a Support Network

Your eco-map can provide a holistic view of your social support system. When you look at an individual's role in your social support system, you can make determinations about who you can go to for help. Now fill in a new eco-map and list both the resources and the individuals in each area that create a positive emotional climate.

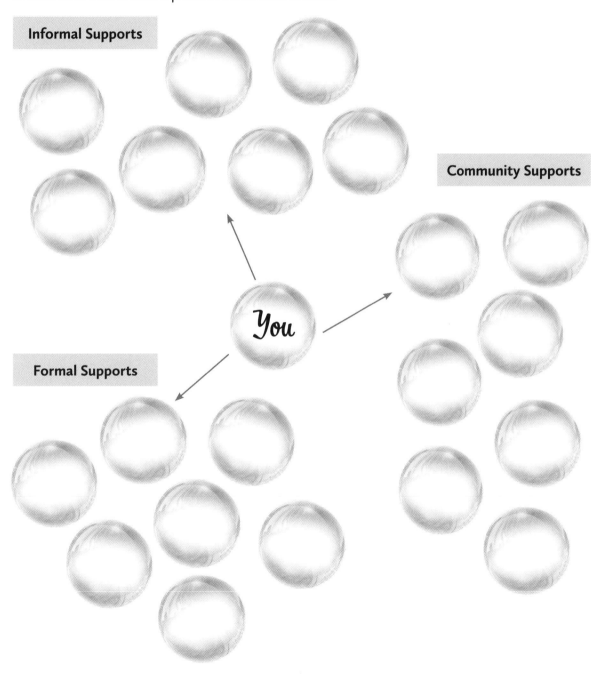

Resourcing Our Social Supports

The next step is looking at how we build or rebuild resources to break down barriers so we can create what we need from our social support systems. To do so, we must recognize those things in our environments that influence our approaches to self-stewardship. Think about these:

- *nuggets* that *nudge* us into self-stewardship practices
- *pushes* that *pull* us from self-stewardship in our personal and professional practices

We did some of this work in chapter 5 when we identified barriers. We want to remember that as we look at barriers, we also look at the resource and supports too. We looked a little at this when we created our eco-maps earlier in the chapter. Let's revisit that now by reflecting on the revised eco-map and making notes on any barriers from activity 5.2 that are preventing us from accessing support. Next we want to identify who is helpful in our eco-map by identifying our support system and mentors.

Build a support system: Look for ways you can add more supports or better supports to your support system. For example, maybe you have a support who provides you with information about your job, but you could benefit from information about the profession outside of your workplace. Maybe you need someone to listen to your feelings about your work, and your current supports just don't acknowledge your needs. We identified needs or holes in our support system. Making a list of supports we need helps us look for and add individuals to our network who can meet specific needs.

Seek out a self-stewardship mentor: Find someone who does self-stewardship well and ask them to help you. If you notice someone who seems to have balance, who can self-regulate their emotions during tense moments, and who upholds the Code of Ethical Conduct, they might be a great mentor. When you approach the mentor, you might begin with a specific question, such as, "I notice that you seem to balance responding to families' concerns while also making time for your own family in the evenings. Can you tell me how you do that?" If you do not have a specific issue in mind, and instead are just overwhelmed, you can approach this possible mentor with a request such as, "I am looking for a mentor, someone who has been doing this job for a while and seems to thrive. Would you be willing to meet with me to discuss how you navigate this work? I would appreciate learning from you."

Mapping our support systems allows us to see the strength and types of our relationships and to consider what each relationship contributes to our well-being. Eco-maps also reveal any gaps we might have in our support structures. We can build our support networks by forming, strengthening, and maintaining relationships with others.

Reflection on Practice

Let's review the questions from the beginning of the chapter.

What do we need to know to navigate our emotional work?

How do our emotional connections build our social support system?

How do we identify our support system resources?

How do we build our social supports?

CHAPTER 8

Building Strong Interpersonal Professional Skills

Interpersonal skills are the competencies that support us in effective interaction with others. The personal attributes and qualities that enable us to successfully navigate our work environments.

We often think of professional skills as those we need in order to teach children. However, professional skills go well beyond how and what we teach and include being in relationship with others and interacting effectively using our interpersonal skills. Strong interpersonal skills include emotional intelligence, interpersonal communication skills, and social abilities that support relationships and collaboration in early childhood classrooms and programs. In this chapter, we ask the following questions:

- What are interpersonal professional skills?
- Why is emotional intelligence important in our daily lives?
- What do strong communication and listening skills look like?
- How do we build strong trusting and healthy relationships?

Professional Interpersonal Skills

Interpersonal skills are the personal attributes and qualities that enable us to navigate our work environments and interact effectively with others. Adaptability, teamwork, time management, conflict resolution, dependability, patience, and leadership are all part of the interpersonal skill set that allow us to be supportive, respectful, kind, engaged, and empathetic. Strong interpersonal skills help us to adjust our approaches to successfully engage others, we also need to be able to navigate the challenges and stressors in our work and engage in self-stewardship.

For the purposes of this workbook, we will focus on three skills that closely align with our work together:

- **Emotional intelligence**—our ability to recognize and manage our emotions as well as the emotions of others.
- **Interpersonal communication skills**—our ability both to communicate our ideas effectively and to listen with care to both verbal and nonverbal feedback.
- **Social abilities**—our ability to build strong, trusting, and healthy relationships.

Emotional Intelligence

Emotional intelligence is our ability to identify, evaluate, and navigate our own and others' emotions. It includes controlling our emotional responses and accurately identifying and addressing others' emotions so we can interpret complex emotions and accurately respond. Our ability to regulate our emotions and the emotions of those around us (children and adults) helps create positive emotional experiences and outcomes.

When we use emotional intelligence, we are able to navigate both positive and negative emotions. This helps us form positive and healthy relationships with friends and colleagues, to navigate the complex emotions of parents, and to regulate ourselves so we can regulate our classrooms, to name a few examples.

Emotional intelligence is generally divided into five skills, two of which—self-awareness and self-regulation—were covered in chapter 4. These are the other three:

- **Social skills**—navigating interactions with others by applying and interpreting our own emotions and those of others, using complex emotional vocabularies to convey a wide variety of emotions, active listening, and developing relationships.
- **Empathy**—perceiving others' emotions and responding accordingly and recognizing the social or power dynamics in a group or workplace. It involves connecting to others' emotions and being open to their life experiences and points of view.
- **Intrinsic motivation**—looking inward rather than outward for validation of our work and being reflective and able to immerse ourselves in our work.

You likely have experienced times when your ability to be emotionally intelligent ebbs and flows throughout your workday, for example, when your intrinsic motivation is strong but self-awareness is challenging. There may be reasons for these shifts that have to do with your environment, schedule, and context. As you continue to build your ability to recognize stress, it can be helpful to notice the moments in the day when emotional work is easy and when it is more challenging.

Mapping Emotional Intelligence and Emotional Energy

Knowing when you have high and low emotional energy is critical to making choices about when you engage in complex emotional work. In this first part of the activity, start by thinking about all you accomplish in your day. Write down the general activities you complete during a workday. Start with the first hour that you are awake, and end with the hour you go to bed.

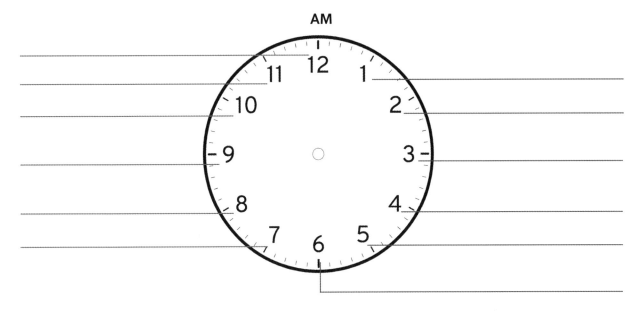

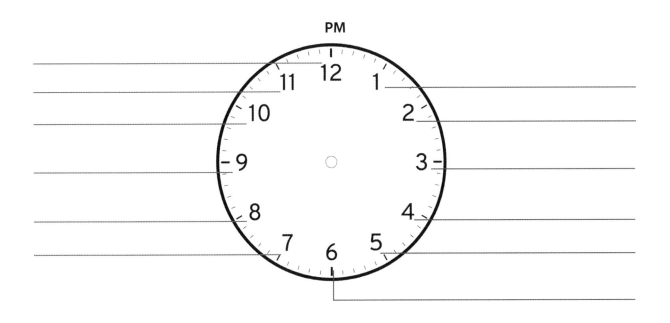

Next, graph your emotional energy during a typical day. Fill in the hour on the bottom line of the following graph (x-axis).

Finally, chart your emotional highs and lows during the day (y-axis). Your energy ebbs and flows as a natural part of your biological clock.

Example

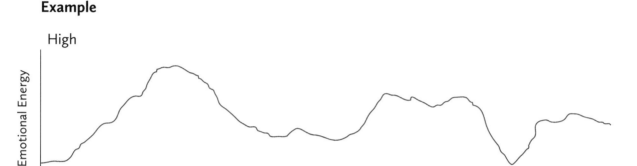

Wake __7 am__ __9 am__ __12 pm__ __3 pm__ __6 pm__ __9 pm__ __11 pm__ Sleep

Here is a graph for you to fill in.

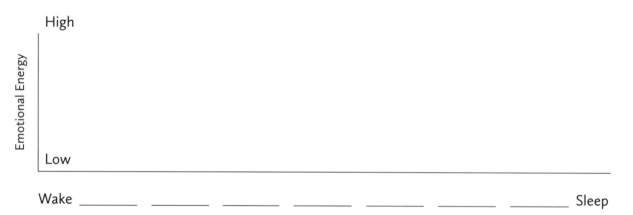

Wake _____ _____ _____ _____ _____ _____ _____ Sleep

By matching activities to our emotional energy, we can see which parts of the day are better for complex conversations, simple tasks, focused attention, and so on. We can pay attention to the ups and downs of our day to acknowledge when we are prepared to engage with others and when we need time alone. Activities like these help us strengthen the five skills of emotional intelligence.

Interpersonal Communication Skills

Strong interpersonal communication involves both sharing and receiving information, with all parties assuming positive intentions from the exchange. It starts with having the ability to express ideas concisely and clearly. The concise expression of ideas demonstrates that we respect the other person enough to take the time to organize and present our thoughts.

Another key skill of interpersonal communication is active listening. Active listening involves listening not only to the words but also to the emotions behind the communication. Active listening means not thinking of your response while the other person is speaking, but instead demonstrate respect for others' beliefs, opinions, and emotions, even when different from your own. For example, if a colleague says something you strongly disagree with, rather than becoming upset, angry, or hurt, pause and consider how you want to respond before acting. Consider your ethical responsibility to young children and use your emotional intelligence to support productive communication between yourself and others. Here is one example. Notice Teacher 1's internal dialogue before responding to Teacher 2. Pausing to reflect before responding is another interpersonal communication skill.

Teacher 1: "Do you know where the paint is? I wanted the children to practice mixing colors."
Teacher 2: "I don't want the children to paint. It is too messy without a sink in the classroom, so I put away all the paint, and I really don't want to do that activity anymore."
Teacher 1 (internal dialogue): I did not agree to put the paint away. It makes me frustrated when decisions are made about important work in the classroom without having a conversation. Ugh! How do I frame my thinking so we can have a successful day and have a conversation later? I want to make sure that I do not start an argument about the paint. But I know paint is an important experience for young children. Let me think about how I can communicate that we need to make decisions together as a team, without making paint a power struggle and affecting how we teach today.
Teacher 1: "Making choices about the paint is a big decision that affects all teachers. I hear concerns about the mess paint can make. I can agree not to put the paint out today. I want to talk about this before we go home because we need to decide together what our next steps are."

Let's look at how the conversation reflects strong interpersonal communication.

- *"Making choices about the paint is a big decision that affects all teachers."* This statement addresses the larger issue of one person making big decisions that affect children and teachers without input.

- *"I hear concerns about the mess paint can make."* This acknowledges the other teacher's reason for this choice and lets Teacher 2 know that the concern was heard and acknowledged.

- *"I can agree not to put the paint out today."* This neutralizes the potential power struggle in the classroom by not trying to solve the problem while the children are waiting to start an activity. Further, Teacher 1 does not feed any of the emotions or power play tactics that Teacher 2 used to push their agenda.
- *"I want to talk about this before we go home because we need to decide together what our next steps are."* Teacher 1 knows that they cannot let the topic go. It is too important. However, it's not the time and place to have the conversation. She is also aware that she does not want to spend a lot of energy on the topic while she is working with the children. So she chooses a response that is neutral but focused.

Based on this brief scenario, we can see how Teacher 1 used their own combination of emotional intelligence, professional ethics, and communication to make decisions for her own professional practice. Teacher 1 cannot control the other teacher but can control her own response and practice her own self-regulation. In doing this, Teacher 1 pays attention to her own emotions, establishes boundaries, works toward modeling healthy relationships, and protects herself from emotional dysregulation.

Communication Scripts

Following communication scripts such as the one described in the scenario can help us build communication skills. They are especially helpful when we prepare for difficult conversations about challenging topics that are likely to result in emotional reactions. It may be tempting to avoid conversations that we know will result in emotional reactions, but these conversations are crucial to resolving conflict, conveying potentially unwanted information, and improving relationships. Taking a moment to notice what might be keeping you from these crucial conversations is an important step in building your communication skills.

Sometimes one of the biggest concerns we have in conflict is the fear of being told no. It may be helpful to recognize that a "no" response can be a protective mechanism when someone feels challenged, overwhelmed, or fearful. Instead of responding in the emotion of the moment, it can be helpful to see an automatic "no" as a time to pause and reflect. Whether you are the one saying no or you are hearing no, take a moment to think about the "why" behind the response. Recognizing the beliefs behind our own or others' automatic responses is an important part of building strong communication skills. Awareness markers and scripts help us develop strong pause-button skills that allow us to make decisions about our work without overwhelming ourselves in the moment, strengthening our professional boundaries. It also helps us to navigate others' responses when they say no to us.

Navigating the "No" Answer

In this example of a communication script, we look at how to navigate a "no." You can use this if you are experiencing a "no" response or find yourself giving one.

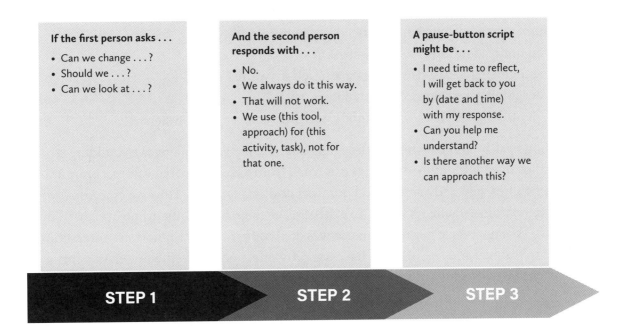

Using the blank template below, to write your own script.

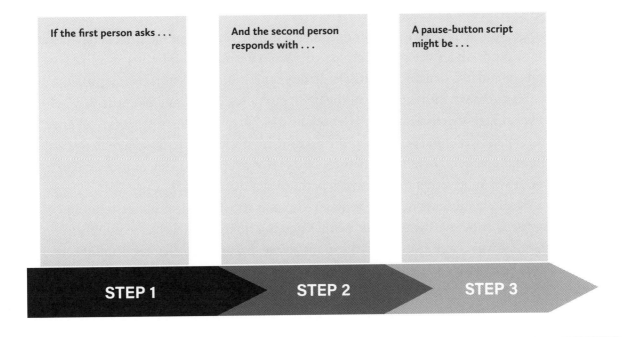

Social Abilities

Strong, trusting, and healthy relationships are a cornerstone of our social abilities. So far in this workbook, we have discussed the many topics that support our ability to build relationships. These include the following:

- a commitment to well-being
- recognizing stress and interpreting our responses to stress
- proactively seeking what we need to promote well-being
- an understanding of self-stewardship
- recognizing demands and barriers to self-stewardship
- developing a strong professional identity
- identifying emotions and building a strong social support system

Building healthy and trusting relationships can be difficult. Challenges to building strong relationships in early childhood settings can come from a lack of shared values, communication difficulties, power dynamics, and our own prior experiences. How we emotionally respond to relational challenges—positive, neutral, or negative—is not evenly weighted in our brains. When we have negative experiences (including thoughts, emotions, interactions, exposure to trauma, and so on), these have a greater effect on our well-being than neutral or positive emotions. Negativity influences how we form impressions about people and situations and how we calculate our sense of risk and safety. It affects how we perceive learning and how we hold memories, which in turn affects our decision-making. For example, when we believe that it is better not to have conflicts with others, we do not share what we think. We may develop coping habits that create unhealthy relationships, like gossiping and having negative conversations about others.

To change, we need to rewire our brains, which is hard work. Our habitual behaviors are like driving a car down a freeway at high speeds. When we rewire our brains, it is like trying to create a road in a dense forest. It takes many repetitions to clear the underbrush, cut down the trees, remove the trunks, level the path, put down gravel, and pave the way before we can move at high speeds again. We fall back into old habits during a process of change because it remains easier to speed down the existing highway than to build a road toward new habits and practices. In building new highways to travel, we also encounter issues that challenge our self-motivation to create new pathways in our brains.

Before we can build these new highways, we must start with a clear understanding of what we need to be successful in our work. Knowing this first allows us to establish boundaries that will foster healthy relationships, as we discussed in chapter 4 about self-stewardship. Boundaries are not about others but rather about what is necessary for our well-being. Sometimes we are tempted to question or shift our boundaries out of fear of others' responses. In these moments, recalling the purpose of boundaries is helpful. Each of us must maintain personal and professional boundaries so that we can be the best versions of ourselves. Building some scripts or responses that allow us to communicate these boundaries to others can be helpful.

Another person's difficulty or inability to recognize and respect your boundary reflects their challenges with self-stewardship, and it's not your problem to solve. Remember that the only person who will always know what you need is you. And in upholding and communicating boundaries in healthy ways, you not only support your own well-being but also model for children how to be healthy in relationships by clearly communicating your needs. Strong self-stewardship means taking the time you need to make the best decision for you. We can adapt activity 8.2 to practice communicating clear professional boundaries.

ACTIVITY 8.3

Communicating Clear Professional Boundaries

Read the script for communicating clear professional boundaries below.

- Listen for the request.
- Consider how you will respond. If you feel a fight, flight, freeze, or fawn response (chapter 3), pause, and answer later.
- If your answer is no, use the script in activity 8.2.
- If you are considering saying yes, do a first appraisal (activity 3.3) and consider the demand and resources needed.

Next, take a few minutes to think about a time when you feel your boundaries felt challenged. Write a brief summary in the space below.

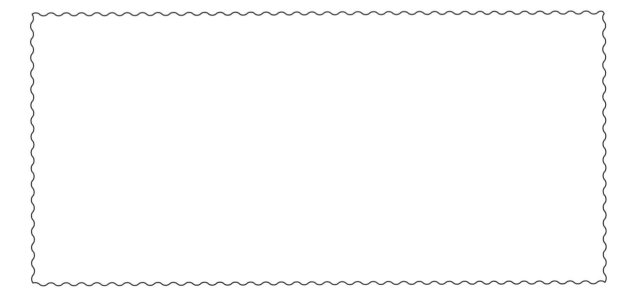

Now let's see how we might reflect on the experience.

Listen for the request.

Consider how you will respond. If you feel a fight, flight, freeze, or fawn response (chapter 3), pause and answer later.

If your answer is no, use the script in activity 8.2.

If you are considering saying yes, do a first appraisal (activity 3.3) and consider the demand and resources needed.

Our interpersonal professional skills help us build and sustain positive healthy relationships. Trust happens over time when we act consistently and with integrity. This chapter focused on the skills we need—emotional intelligence, interpersonal communication skills, and social abilities—to build and sustain trust through our professional practices. Strong interpersonal skills support strong healthy and trusting relationships in early childhood classrooms and programs.

Reflection on Practice

Let's review the questions from the beginning of the chapter.

What are interpersonal professional skills?

Why is emotional intelligence important in our daily lives?

What do strong communication and listening skills look like?

How do we build strong trusting and healthy relationships?

CHAPTER 9

Solving Problems Every Day

Problem solving is the ability to remove or address barriers and resource the problem with appropriate reflective, emotional, or professional skills.

In our final two chapters, we gather all of the reflective practices, emotional work, and professional skills of the previous chapter and turn to problem solving. Problem solving is about identifying barriers and demands and deciding how we use our resources to find solutions that reinforce and do not sacrifice our well-being. We attend to our well-being through daily problem solving, making and reinforcing choices that support our emotional health. In this chapter, we ask the following questions:

- How do we identify problems?
- What is the difference between big and little problems?
- What do we need to believe to solve problems?
- How do we prioritize the problems we solve?

Solving Problems Every Day

The typical workday is filled with problems to solve. It might be as simple as locating an address, finessing the wording of a newsletter item, or figuring out how to copy something when the copier is broken. But the problem also could be something bigger, like talking to a family about a child's developmental delays or asking an administrator about changing the schedule for recess.

Other common problems in early childhood settings can include these:

- talking to a coworker about a disagreement
- responding to the director's request to stay late
- talking to an angry parent
- requesting a raise and having it denied
- handling ongoing staffing shortages or being out of ratio
- facing expectations to take work home

Attending to problems all day is a critical part of the work of early childhood teachers, and it is also draining. Before realizing it, you can become weary—weary of encountering and responding to concerns or of lacking the time to attend to larger questions of interest or to envision something new for yourself and the children and families you serve. Avoiding burnout requires us to identify problems, use robust strategies for solving problems, and understand and respect the emotional work involved in problem solving (Brown et al. 2018).

When facing problems of any kind, we want a sense of control. Making a list and breaking down the challenge is an often-used strategy for gaining a sense of control or allowing reflection. As we turn our attention to stress, emotions, and problem solving, list making may help here too.

Big and Little Problems

One day when Jenny was worrying about some problem, her mentor told her DSTSS, "Don't sweat the small stuff." Apparently, he felt that the challenge she was facing and the stress she was feeling were "small" and therefore insignificant. We tend to categorize problems as "big" and "little" and convince ourselves that we only need to pay attention to the big problems. But any hiccup can feel stressful. And small things can cause big emotions and be important, if only for the way they impact us.

There are problems that we see, but also problems we only *feel*. We may quickly notice the big, obvious obstructions: the boulders. This is helpful as it allows us to prepare, anticipate challenges, and interpret when we are stressed. However, the smaller, nearly invisible issues are like sand that collects in our shoes. We might be able to ignore it for a while, but eventually we'll have blisters from constant rubbing, which will force us to stop walking. Our own contexts and characteristics can determine whether problems, big or little, are positive or dangerous.

Before we can even begin to prioritize what is urgent or important, we need to recognize the problem, and sometimes this work is harder than we think. For example, consider an early childhood teacher who is continually struggling with classroom organization. She finds herself having to regroup and replace items on the shelves every day, spending time returning items back to their place, and this keeps her from being able to leave work on time. While the problem might look like a lack of time, the underlying issue might really be too many items in the room, a lack of clear indicators for where to place things, or even children not being taught how to care for the classroom materials. Spending hours and energy each day pushing through the cleanup work and dealing with the stress related to lost time can keep the teacher too busy to see the underlying issues. The very tools and coping strategies that allow us to keep pressing forward and respond to urgent matters can become the reasons we just don't see a problem.

In this chapter, we will work through activities as a way of reflecting and thinking deeply about solving problems.

Boulders in the Road and Sand in the Shoe

If I were to ask you right now to make a list of the problems you have to solve in your work, could you do it? Some problems might come readily to mind, such as a challenging interaction with a family or a scheduling concern. Whatever comes up first is likely the problem that is causing you the most stress at the moment. Take a few minutes to brainstorm problems that emerge.

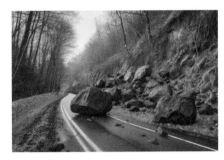

Visible and Obvious Problems (Boulders in the Road)

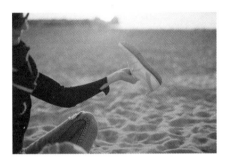

Almost Invisible Everyday Problems (Sand in the Shoe)

Whether a problem is visible and obvious or almost invisible, all problems fall into one of two categories: technical or adaptive (Heifetz and Laurie 1997). **Technical problems** are usually readily identifiable and can be quickly solved with concrete solutions, leaning on existing expertise. Teachers learn how to solve technical problems through training, experience, and observing others. If we have the expertise required, or we at least know something about how to solve the problems, these technical challenges can be experienced like sand: challenging to walk through, seemingly everywhere, and fatiguing, yet with clear solutions. Most of the challenges we face each day fall into the "technical" category.

Adaptive problems require new knowledge or new approaches. These challenges are novel and can be scary because we struggle to identify the problem or lack the knowledge required to solve it. We use adaptive problem solving when we recognize that our existing approaches to problem solving—our technical solutions—don't work. One example of an adaptive challenge in our profession is the concern about having a sufficient number of teachers in a program. As a profession, our traditional approaches for posting jobs are not working. However, if we apply adaptive problem solving to the issue of staffing, we might discover a new approach, such as growing our own teachers.

Categorizing Problems

What categories do your problems fall into?

Technical Problems   **Adaptive Problems**

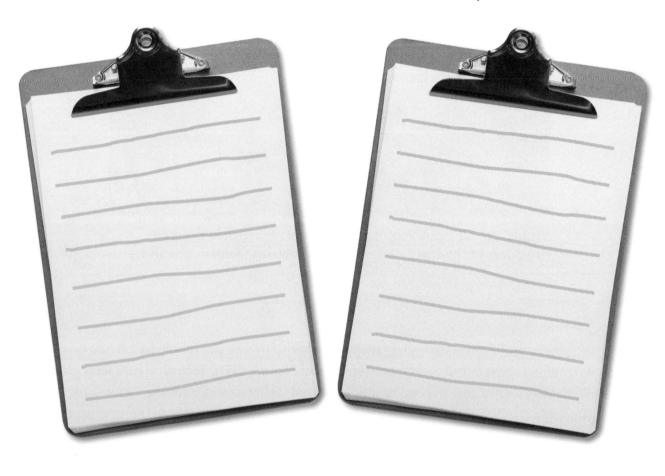

As you are thinking about these big, challenging problems, it can be helpful to realize that you successfully solve many problems daily. The "small stuff" problems likely did not come to mind at first when you were making your lists, but you tackle those all the time. The skills you have for solving "small stuff" problems allow you to solve larger problems too. Remember that you have developed many tools from the first eight chapters of this workbook. These will help you as you tackle bigger, more intimidating problems. Now let's take a moment to look at some of the specific strategies you can use to solve problems.

Strategies for Solving Problems

There is a great deal of advice about problem solving (sometimes called *decision-making*) in the workplace. Most of it presents the steps as very linear and straightforward:

- Determine what the problem or challenge is.
- Brainstorm possible actions to address the problem or challenge.
- Review the benefits and drawbacks of each solution (pros and cons).
- Choose a solution to try.
- Put the solution into action.
- Determine if the solution worked and change or modify the approach as needed.

But this list is not always practical. Sometimes there are no clear options or responses, and sometimes all of the costs seem too high. Sometimes we may not have the power needed to make the decision.

Despite knowing idealized strategies, we often fall into habits of decision-making, wherein we take an easier or more familiar path instead of the optimal one. The following actions are common when we make decisions:

- deciding on a solution based on the first idea that comes to mind
- making decisions based on gut instinct
- letting go and not making a decision
- asking someone else to make the decision
- overanalyzing choices
- being indecisive and changing back and forth between possible solutions
- only choosing safe solutions
- trying to plan for every outcome

Perhaps you spend a lot of time agonizing over a decision, investigating every possible outcome. Another person might be more impulsive, just choosing what seems right at the moment. With this approach to decision-making, problems are at least temporarily solved, but making decisions without additional information or time for reflection can create other problems. Impulsivity is different from an intuitive approach to problem solving, in which a person senses or feels through decisions. Intuitive approaches draw on professional skills, including reflection and observation, to determine a solution. If you tend to put off a decision, you may be playing it safe and avoiding the emotions and thinking involved in making a decision.

Each of us tends to have a go-to strategy for addressing problems. For example, knowing and acknowledging our penchant for delaying can help us be more intentional in our practice and in building our professional skills. In chapter 10, we will introduce a new pathway to help with decision-making. But first, let's look a little at your current approaches. The following activity helps us identify our default strategies for decision-making and problem solving.

Match Actions To Decisions

Look back at the list of problems and decisions (activity 9.2) you face during your workday.

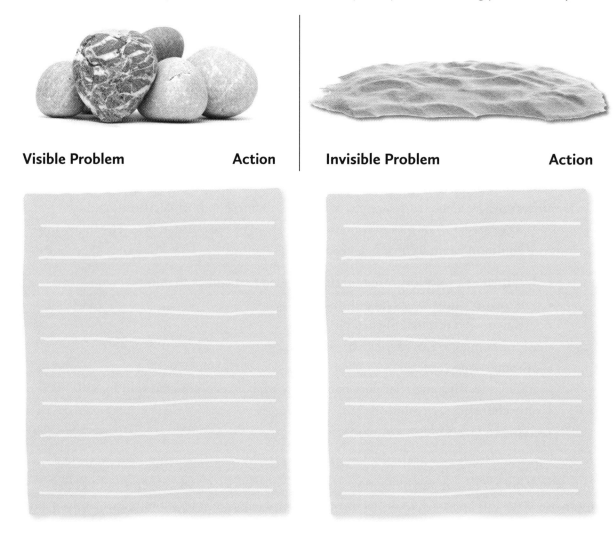

Visible Problem	Action	Invisible Problem	Action

Then reflect on these questions:

- Is there a pattern in my approaches to decisions?
- Is there something I would like to change about the way I solve problems?

Understanding Your Priorities

Big and little problems all require solutions, but not every problem has to be solved immediately, and not every problem has to be solved by you. Determining where to invest your time and energy is a big factor in addressing workplace stress.

One strategy, using the Eisenhower Matrix, sorts problems by urgency and importance. In this approach, we are encouraged to think carefully about the nature of the problem before us. Sometimes everything seems urgent and important. This is when it is helpful to stop and think about the problem clearly.

ACTIVITY 9.4

Determining Which Problems to Solve First

List all the activities you engage in, in a single day. Then place them in the matrix below based on importance and urgency.

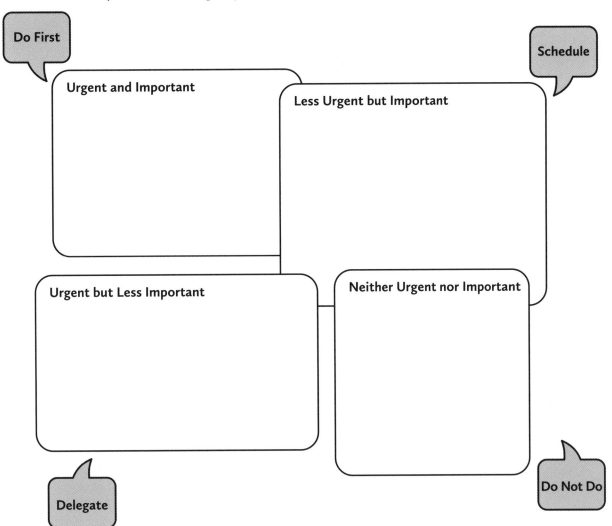

Many people find this matrix helpful when facing a never-ending to-do list or a list of problems to solve. The idea is to think carefully about what is really important and to separate those things from the things that just appear urgent but are not that critical. In other words, we are working on our appraisal of the problem.

The daily work with families, children, and colleagues involves decision-making and problem solving. Sometimes these decisions are invisible and made without much fuss, and other times they are all we can think about. Understanding the nature of the problems we encounter in our work is the first step in unpacking our stress responses. When we correctly identify the importance or lack of importance of a problem, we can sort our demands better and choose where to focus our attention.

Reflection on Practice

Let's review the questions from the beginning of the chapter.

How do we identify problems?

What is the difference between big and little problems?

What do we need to believe to solve problems?

How do we prioritize the problems we solve?

CHAPTER 10

The Problem-Solving Pathway

The Problem-Solving Pathway is a self-stewardship action plan using reflective practices, emotional work, and professional skills to resource demands and solve problems in a way that supports well-being.

You have done so much reflecting, thinking, and processing, and now it is time to talk about how you can use all of this when you go to work tomorrow. While it would be wonderful if we could have a script for every circumstance and a plan for self-stewardship with a 100 percent guarantee of success, the steps for addressing problems and ensuring well-being are not linear. Instead, they are what we call an ***iterative process,*** meaning they involve creating, testing, and refining. In this final chapter, we will present a process and framework to help you in the emotional work of educating and caring for young children. We offer this as a tool for engaging in the self-stewardship we have discussed so often.

We each have a role in ensuring our own well-being. However, systems support—ensuring that the profession of early childhood education supports the well-being of all its members—is also critical in helping each of us imagine, plan, and advocate for change. In this chapter, we ask the following questions:

- How do we solve problems every day?
- How might we use the Problem-Solving Pathway?
- How does the Problem-Solving Pathway support self-stewardship?
- How does the Problem-Solving Pathway support well-being?

The Problem-Solving Pathway for Well-Being

The **Problem-Solving Pathway** (Baumgartner and Anderson 2021) was designed to help you practice leadership by giving you resources for making decisions every day that promote well-being. While you will find many books and resources related to professional problem solving, the Problem-Solving Pathway recognizes that emotional work is also necessary to navigate the big and small problems that arise every day in early childhood classrooms, as is attending to our well-being.

When we are unsure about how to solve a problem, the Problem-Solving Pathway supports us in accessing the reflective and professional skills we need to emotionally finesse the work—in other words, to be good self-stewards. While this pathway is presented as a linear series of steps and questions, please know there will be times on our journey when encountering something new demands that we turn and revisit a previous step along the way. And because this is not a test, we offer some hints alongside the questions. Let's get started.

The Questions We Ask in Supporting Our Self-Stewardship

1. What is the problem I am experiencing at this moment? *Hint: See chapter 3.*

As you have worked through this book, several problems or demands have likely surfaced. In chapters 3 and 9, you even worked at naming some of these. To use the pathway, start by thinking about a problem or demand you are experiencing and name it. As we have discussed throughout the book, this step can be powerful. Moving the problem from one you only feel to one you can think about is critical. Remember too that there might be demands and challenges that are less obvious. Here are some questions you might ask as you ponder the problem or demand:

- What am I being asked to do?
- Is it a direct demand, request, or requirement of my job (in my job description, as a licensing requirement, or something else)?
- Is it understood to be part of my work but not explicitly written?
- Who is telling me that I need to do this?

Our professional environments are filled with requirements, ideas, cultures, expectations, and ideals that influence what we do as teachers and how we do it. Sometimes we only "sense" a problem, or we find ourselves behaving in ways that are inconsistent with our professional identities (the kind of people we believe ourselves to be).

2. What is my first appraisal of the problem? *Hint: Look at chapter 3.*

After you have identified the demand, the scary part of recognizing and labeling the emotions that come with it is next. You may recall from our earlier discussion that stress can be an indicator of an unmet need. It is important to pay attention to the somatic symptoms that indicate a challenging emotion. Some frequently mentioned symptoms include stomach pains, fatigue, dizziness, and tearfulness. Think of it as a warning signal in your car. If we continue driving as normal, ignoring the signal or the symptoms, we can expect damage.

Consider the problem you identified in step 1 and notice the emotions that come up. Be careful not to assign any value or judgment to the emotions. This is a time for noticing only.

- Where am I experiencing stress (in my body, mind, or both)?
- What stage of stress am I experiencing (alarm, resistance, exhaustion, and so on)?
- Do I experience fight, flight, freeze, or fawn responses?
- What tend to be my first coping responses?

3. What might be keeping me from practicing self-stewardship? *Hint: See chapter 4.*

It takes work to notice and address how you lead yourself through your self-stewardship practices. In a job that has countless demands, it is often easier just to turn to the next urgent task than make choices based on your professional identity in keeping with the NAEYC Code of Ethical Conduct. But as you pursue well-being and engage in self-stewardship, stop and think about your natural tendencies for handling decision-making. As discussed earlier, you probably have go-to ways of coping with stress. Think about how you are coping and setting boundaries with this particular problem or demand. Is it in keeping with your goals of self-stewardship? Here are some questions that might help you with your processing:

- What is my process for checking the NAEYC Code of Ethical Conduct?
- How do I make decisions on my professional values and beliefs?
- What boundaries am I setting for myself?
- How am I practicing self-stewardship?

4. What are the demands and barriers I am facing? *Hint: See chapter 5.*

Getting stopped on the journey to well-being is a common occurrence. Sometimes you'll encounter an obvious roadblock, such as a crisis or an interruption that requires (demands) your focus. However, perpetually responding to crises without self-stewardship is unsustainable. There may be barriers in your context that keep you from fully caring for yourself.

- Do I have the resources to meet the demand?
- If not, what are the barriers that I am facing in meeting the demand?
- Are the barriers external or internal?
- What barriers impede my efforts to practice self-stewardship?

5. How can I access my toolbox? *Hint: See chapters 6 and 7.*

Now is the time to access your toolbox, drawing from chapter 6, which you use to strengthen your professional identity. Acknowledging your strengths and limitations and seeking supports are part of filling your toolbox. Use chapter 7 to identify and access resources for your emotional work. Then adapt the skills in chapter 8 to plan your interpersonal engagement to access supports.

6. How can I connect to my professional identity? *Hint: See chapter 6.*

Sometimes a demand or problem makes sense, meaning it fits the job duties and typical assignments of the job. Others are outside of the professional scope. For those that are a part of your professional practice, the request or demand can reinforce our sense of self-respect, agency, contribution, and security. However, demands that are outside of the professional scope serve to decrease these qualities. Finally, some demands are harmful and dangerous. These occur if you are asked to compromise your professional practice. In other words, it is not what you are supposed to be doing.

Starting with the NAEYC Code of Ethical Conduct ensures that you are looking at the problem within the context of your professional practice. The code will guide you in determining what is in the best interest of children, families, and colleagues. It will guide your ethical decision-making. Many problems have clear guidelines in the Code of Ethical Conduct.

- Is there anything about this problem that is challenging my professional identity?
- What guidance does the Code of Ethical Conduct provide?
- How do I use my professional commitment to center my professional identity on problem solving?
- How am I identifying professional wellness practices to help me make decisions?

7. How do I develop my support system? *Hint: See chapter 7.*

Now let's think about the resources and supports that are available to you as you work to meet this demand. Because emotions are a part of the work of meeting demands, you will want to make sure you have emotional supports who can help you as you navigate through this process. Reflecting on the resources and sources of support in your life—the people and groups who can help you specifically with the demand you have outlined—is a critical part of the process.

Here are some questions to consider as you think about the path forward:

- Do I have the resources I need to address this problem?
- If I do, what is stopping me from using them in this way?
- If I don't, how can I access these resources?
- If there are no resources available to me to address this demand, can I eliminate or reframe the demand?

8. How do I plan my interactions to solve the problem? *Hint: See chapter 8.*

After identifying the support you need, it is time to engage your interpersonal professional skills to access that support in ways that will help you meet the demand. Using your emotional intelligence to recognize your emotions and those of others will help you engage in more focused and productive forms of communication that will support your ability to meet the demand.

- How does what I know about emotions—mine and others—help me as I address this demand?
- How can I effectively and productively communicate about this demand? How might my use of scripts help me plan for a productive conversation?
- What relationships are critical to me? How can I ensure that these remain strong or are even improved?
- What boundaries do I need to maintain?

9. How can I build well-being into my decision-making? *Hint: See chapter 9.*

It is one thing to set a goal of wellness. It is another to have this goal at the forefront of decision-making. When you experience problems or demands, finding a solution is compelling, and counting the personal cost to well-being often comes late, if it is considered at all. The goal of this pathway is to bring wellness front and center in your processing. There are times when you will experience demands that are inconsistent with this goal of wellness. In these cases, it may be necessary to make difficult choices that uphold your own well-being. Here are some questions and ideas to consider when making these evaluations:

- What are my top priorities in my work each day? Is well-being on the list?
- Do I have others around me who support and reinforce my goals for well-being?
- Do I understand what well-being means for me personally? Do I know when I am well and when I am unwell?
- Do I have a plan of action to make sure that wellness remains a priority? Are there accountability checks and moments for me to realize when I have slipped in prioritizing this?

Misidentifying what we need to address the demands placed on us decreases our creativity, curiosity, and motivation. Like children, adults who practice multiple problem-solving strategies enhance their sense of empowerment, agency, and self-stewardship. Remember that no one masters new ways of appraising demands overnight. It takes time to learn new patterns of thinking and to rewire our brains. Let's look at some ways to begin.

Building Your Problem-Solving Pathway

The Problem-Solving Pathway brings all the steps of the book together as you engage in self-stewardship to support your well-being. The decisions you need to make every day are the ones that most affect your well-being. The Problem-Solving Pathway examples illustrate how this tool works.

The Problem-Solving Pathway

By Jennifer J. Baumgartner and Ingrid Mari Anderson

Some problems are easy to solve, but some leave you feeling unsure. Self-stewardship is about understanding and addressing your emotional well-being. Use the Problem-Solving Pathway to identify the demands and the resources you need to meet those demands. Use the pathway to address stress and choose proactive coping strategies.

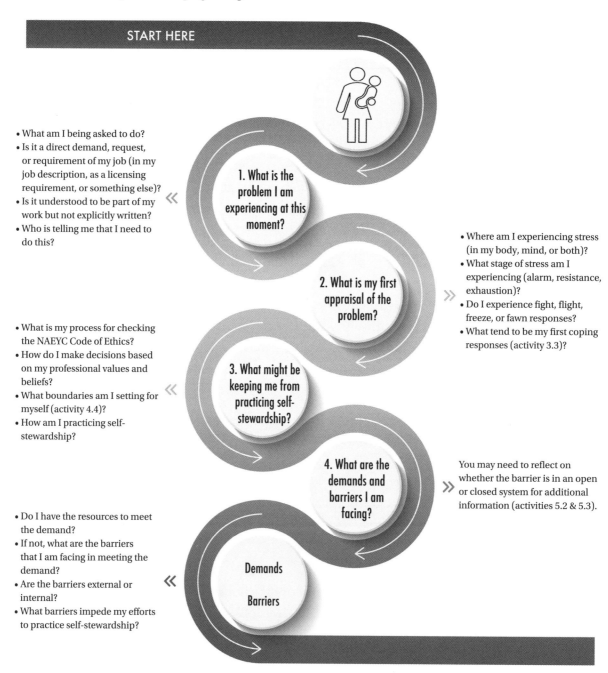

START HERE

- What am I being asked to do?
- Is it a direct demand, request, or requirement of my job (in my job description, as a licensing requirement, or something else)?
- Is it understood to be part of my work but not explicitly written?
- Who is telling me that I need to do this?

1. What is the problem I am experiencing at this moment?

2. What is my first appraisal of the problem?

- Where am I experiencing stress (in my body, mind, or both)?
- What stage of stress am I experiencing (alarm, resistance, exhaustion)?
- Do I experience fight, flight, freeze, or fawn responses?
- What tend to be my first coping responses (activity 3.3)?

- What is my process for checking the NAEYC Code of Ethics?
- How do I make decisions based on my professional values and beliefs?
- What boundaries am I setting for myself (activity 4.4)?
- How am I practicing self-stewardship?

3. What might be keeping me from practicing self-stewardship?

4. What are the demands and barriers I am facing?

You may need to reflect on whether the barrier is in an open or closed system for additional information (activities 5.2 & 5.3).

- Do I have the resources to meet the demand?
- If not, what are the barriers that I am facing in meeting the demand?
- Are the barriers external or internal?
- What barriers impede my efforts to practice self-stewardship?

Demands

Barriers

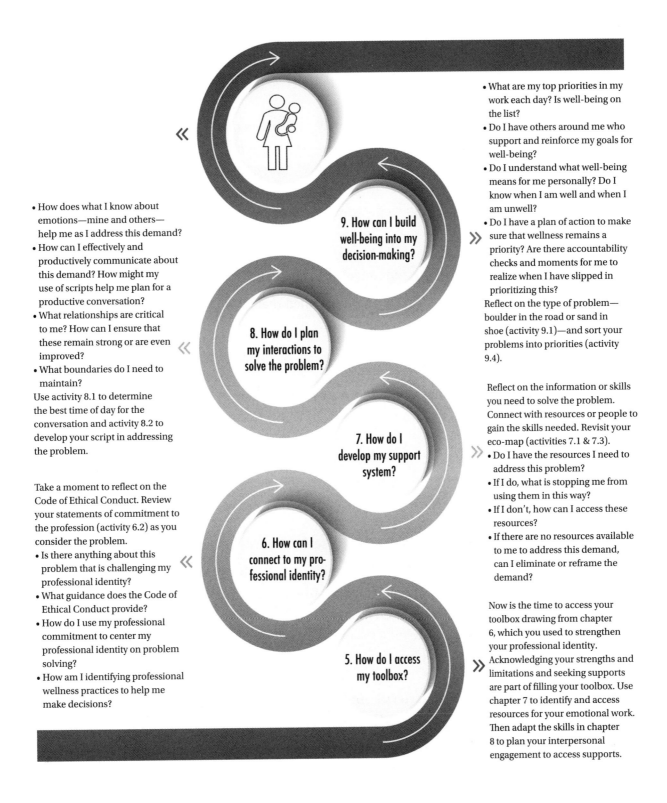

- How does what I know about emotions—mine and others—help me as I address this demand?
- How can I effectively and productively communicate about this demand? How might my use of scripts help me plan for a productive conversation?
- What relationships are critical to me? How can I ensure that these remain strong or are even improved?
- What boundaries do I need to maintain?

Use activity 8.1 to determine the best time of day for the conversation and activity 8.2 to develop your script in addressing the problem.

Take a moment to reflect on the Code of Ethical Conduct. Review your statements of commitment to the profession (activity 6.2) as you consider the problem.

- Is there anything about this problem that is challenging my professional identity?
- What guidance does the Code of Ethical Conduct provide?
- How do I use my professional commitment to center my professional identity on problem solving?
- How am I identifying professional wellness practices to help me make decisions?

9. How can I build well-being into my decision-making?

8. How do I plan my interactions to solve the problem?

7. How do I develop my support system?

6. How can I connect to my professional identity?

5. How do I access my toolbox?

- What are my top priorities in my work each day? Is well-being on the list?
- Do I have others around me who support and reinforce my goals for well-being?
- Do I understand what well-being means for me personally? Do I know when I am well and when I am unwell?
- Do I have a plan of action to make sure that wellness remains a priority? Are there accountability checks and moments for me to realize when I have slipped in prioritizing this?

Reflect on the type of problem—boulder in the road or sand in shoe (activity 9.1)—and sort your problems into priorities (activity 9.4).

Reflect on the information or skills you need to solve the problem. Connect with resources or people to gain the skills needed. Revisit your eco-map (activities 7.1 & 7.3).

- Do I have the resources I need to address this problem?
- If I do, what is stopping me from using them in this way?
- If I don't, how can I access these resources?
- If there are no resources available to me to address this demand, can I eliminate or reframe the demand?

Now is the time to access your toolbox drawing from chapter 6, which you used to strengthen your professional identity. Acknowledging your strengths and limitations and seeking supports are part of filling your toolbox. Use chapter 7 to identify and access resources for your emotional work. Then adapt the skills in chapter 8 to plan your interpersonal engagement to access supports.

We now apply the Problem-Solving Pathway to a real example in early childhood education.

Self-Stewardship in Action

Jerri is a preschool teacher at a nonprofit community child care center. The center and the staff enjoy a good reputation in the community, and the director is invested in creating a learning environment that is responsive to children's and teachers' interests. While Jerri receives support in some areas, her direct supervisor seems to dismiss Jerri when Jerri says that she is stressed or frustrated in her work. Overall, Jerri feels isolated and unsupported. She is hesitant to go over her supervisor's head to the director because she does not want to rock the boat or cause problems.

How can Jerri use the Problem-Solving Pathway to better understand what she needs to do next?

What is the problem I am experiencing at this moment?

Jerri feels isolated and unsupported. She is concerned that approaching the director will cause problems between her and the supervisor.

What is my first appraisal of the problem?

Jerri is anxious when she thinks about addressing this problem. She is scared about "rocking the boat" and stepping out. One moment she feels conviction and wants to do something, and other times she wonders, "What if I just stay quiet? What if my director gets mad at me for complaining about my supervisor?" Noticing these emotions, especially those that are in conflict, is an important part of the process for her. She decides that the way to handle the emotions is to address the problem she has identified.

What might be keeping me from practicing self-stewardship?

When Jerri stops to think about how she is handling the problem, she realizes that she is not taking action. Rather than stepping forward to solve the problem, she is avoiding interactions with her supervisor by not even going to the break room to get her normal cup of coffee. Instead, she eats chocolate in her room when she needs a pick-me-up. She complains about her supervisor to her spouse at home every night.

What are the demands and barriers I am facing?

When Jerri thinks through what is stopping her, she realizes that she has concerns about retaliation and her employment. She also is afraid that confronting this issue will make everyone uncomfortable and may cause her to lose friends. She realizes that she would like to increase her positive emotions about work.

How can I access my toolbox?

Jerri considers why she feels unsupported. She realizes that she is uncomfortable with the discrepancy between what her director says and what her supervisor does. Jerri realizes that she needs to make a plan to move forward by accessing her toolbox. This problem involves actions she takes as a professional, understanding both strengths and limitations of her current skills, and finding the emotional supports she needs to plan her engagement with the individuals involved.

How can I connect to my professional identity?

Jerri realizes that her fear comes from not checking in with herself and her professional values and beliefs. She realizes that she is not consulting the NAEYC Code of Ethical Conduct when considering solutions. She considers how the Code could help her with language to determine what to say as the concern is about professional actions at work. Using the Code supports a conversation on professional practices in the workplace and skill building.

How do I develop my support system?

When Jerri thinks about moving forward, she realizes that she could address this issue if she had some help dealing with the negative emotions she has toward her supervisor, and if she knew more about handling conflict.

How do I plan my interactions to solve the problem?

Jerri makes a plan so that she can take care of herself as she moves through the process of addressing this issue and others to come. First, she realizes that she will need to meet with her director. She recognizes that she needs people to support her as she solves the problem. She also realizes that she needs some tools for handling conflict with superiors. She finds a good book on the subject and connects with a mentor who can help her practice these skills.

How can I build well-being into my decision-making?

To increase her positive emotions when engaged in work, Jerri decides to set up regular coffee breaks with a colleague who is cheerful and thoughtful. Finally, to help her keep in touch with her emotions that might lead to avoidance and discontent, Jerri starts to journal each night, recording her thoughts and feelings about the day.

Completing Your Own Pathway

It is your turn to try the Problem-Solving Pathway. Start by reflecting on the questions below.

- What is the problem I am experiencing at this moment?
- What is my first appraisal of the problem?
- What might be keeping me from practicing self-stewardship?
- What are the demands and barriers I am facing?
- How can I access my toolbox?
- How can I connect to my professional identity?
- How do I develop my support system?
- How do I plan my interactions to solve the problem?
- How can I build well-being into my decision-making?

Next, use the blank pathway to solve a problem by filling in the boxes. You can refer back to the details in the figure on pages 104–105 if you become stuck at any step in the process. See blank Problem Solving Pathway on pages 110–111.

Conclusion

Your well-being is important—not just because of the impact you have on the children and families, but because *you* are important. As an early childhood teacher, you have leadership skills you can direct toward ensuring your own well-being. Self-stewardship protects your physical, social, cognitive, emotional, psychological, and spiritual self by helping you accurately categorize, appraise, and resource the demands you face.

However, you are not the only one responsible for wellness in early childhood. As we look at our profession riddled with stress and burnout of its members, it is obvious that early childhood systems need to do a better job of engaging with teachers to make sure they have the resources they need. There are systematic changes that can and should be made to ensure the well-being of all who are a part of the profession. The first step to advocating for these changes is to make sure you are well. We cannot wait for others to help us make the proactive choices we need to have healthy lives. It is up to us to lead ourselves and to act with self-compassion, holding strong professional boundaries for our own well-being.

Reflection on Practice

Let's review the questions from the beginning of the chapter.

How do we solve problems every day?	How might we use the Problem-Solving Pathway?

How does the Problem-Solving Pathway support self-stewardship?	How does the Problem-Solving Pathway support well-being?

The Problem-Solving Pathway

By Jennifer J. Baumgartner and Ingrid Mari Anderson

Some problems are easy to solve, but some leave you feeling unsure. Self-stewardship is about understanding and addressing your emotional well-being. Use the Problem-Solving Pathway to identify the demands and the resources you need to meet those demands. Use the pathway to address stress and choose proactive coping strategies.

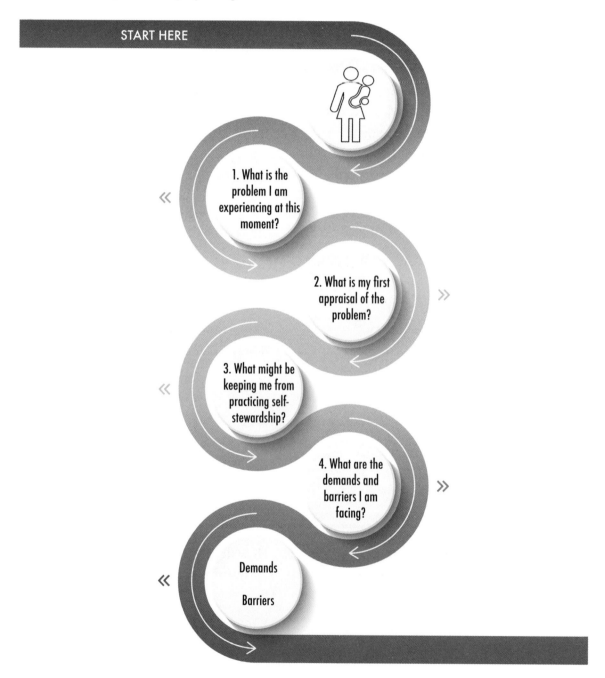

START HERE

1. What is the problem I am experiencing at this moment?

2. What is my first appraisal of the problem?

3. What might be keeping me from practicing self-stewardship?

4. What are the demands and barriers I am facing?

Demands

Barriers

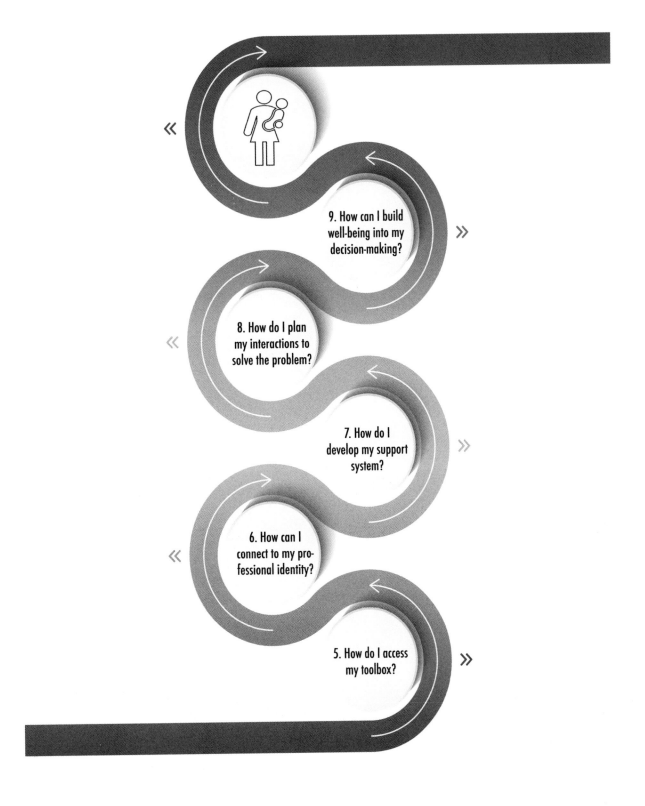

9. How can I build well-being into my decision-making?

8. How do I plan my interactions to solve the problem?

7. How do I develop my support system?

6. How can I connect to my professional identity?

5. How do I access my toolbox?

GLOSSARY

adaptive problem: A problem that requires new knowledge or a new approach. These challenges are novel and can be scary because a person may struggle to understand the problem or lack the knowledge required to solve it.

altruism: A form of selflessness that can mean sacrificing one's own personal well-being for others.

appraisal: A cognitive process of assessing the degree of danger. It can serve as a form of triage.

barrier: An obstacle to our self-stewardship.

being in care of self: The ongoing practice of taking responsibility for one's own physical, emotional, cognitive, social, psychological, and spiritual needs through mindful practices.

belonging: Community-based support that is organized around a sense of belonging or place. Support can come from an informal group of individuals or a larger, more formal organization.

boundary: A line that defines one area from another. In the context of relationships, a boundary is a limit a person places on themselves regarding what they will and will not do.

burnout: A state of exhaustion that can occur across physical, emotional, cognitive, social, psychological, and/or spiritual domains.

closed system: A system that may be under-resourced or feature an uneven distribution of resources. Closed early childhood systems are isolated and self-contained.

cognitive well-being: One's mental flexibility and imagination.

community support: An organization in one's community that provides support, such as a club or spiritual home.

complex emotions: Nuanced adaptations of emotions—part of our conscious thought—that we interpret to respond to the world around us.

coping: The strategies (physical, emotional, cognitive, social, psychological, or spiritual) that we use to adapt and handle experiences and challenges.

defense response: A natural reaction to the demands placed on the body from physically, mentally, and cognitively challenging situations. Alarm, resistance, and exhaustion are the three stages of physiological and psychological reaction to stress.

demand: A requirement or need that must be met.

eco-map: A graphic representation tool created by Ann Hartman. A map or drawing depicts an individual's informal, formal, and intermediate supports.

emotional health: One's capacity to develop, understand, express, and navigate a wide range of human emotions (at developmentally appropriate levels) and to recognize and respond to the emotions in others.

emotional support: People who provide support for emotions, including recognizing and validating emotions. Emotional supports also include individuals who help us laugh, lift our moods, or increase our sense of positivity.

emotional well-being: The quality of one's emotional responses to life experiences, including one's ability to adapt and change, demonstrate resiliency, resolve conflicts, manage emotions, and generate consistent feelings of happiness and hopefulness.

emotional work: The process of identifying, accessing, and applying tools to navigate emotions and build relationships that support well-being.

empathy: An ability to understand others' emotions and respond accordingly. Empathy includes the ability to recognize the social or power dynamics in a group or workplace. It involves connecting to others' emotions and being open to their life experiences and points of view.

external barrier: Something outside of oneself that prevents self-stewardship and wellness.

fawn: A defense response that involves pleasing others to avoid conflict.

fight: A defense response that uses aggressive behaviors to address a threat. This can include physical, emotional, social, or cognitive responses.

flight: A defense response that involves removing oneself from a perceived danger physically, emotionally, socially, or cognitively.

formal support: A formal relationship created with a primary goal of providing support. Formal supports include medical care providers, counselors, and human resource managers.

freeze: A defense response that involves being unable to act against a threat.

informal support: A source of support that is not formally defined, such as from a family member, friend, or neighbor.

informational support: A support who shares information—including advice and ideas—and instruction. An informational support may help us learn something new in our work or identify a resource for us.

instrumental support: Support that includes assistance in physical ways (this can be someone who gives us a ride when our car doesn't start, helps us move, or sets up an area of the classroom for us). Instrumental supports are generally focused on practice or tangible supports in our everyday lives.

internal barrier: A barrier that you carry that keeps you from self-stewardship. Some common examples are guilt or feeling unworthy.

interpersonal skills: Skills that support us in effective interaction with others. The personal attributes and qualities that enable us to successfully navigate our work environments.

intrinsic motivation: Leading oneself in one's work. Looking inward rather than outward for validation of one's work. Being reflective and able to immerse oneself in their work.

iterative process: A process that involves creation, testing, and refining.

limbic system: The part of the brain that makes decisions based on emotion and impulse.

NAEYC Code of Ethics: Are published by the National Association for the Education of Young Children and are the professional principles for the early childhood profession that guide professional practice.

open system: A system with open boundaries that create transparency between members of the early childhood community—educators, families, and children.

physical well-being: The care of the physical body, including sleep, healthy eating, hydration, personal health (medical and dental), and personal care.

problem-solving: The ability to remove or address barriers and resource the problem with appropriate reflective, emotional, or professional skills.

The Problem-Solving Pathway: A self-stewardship action plan using reflective practices, emotional work, and professional skills to resource demands and solve problems in a way that supports well-being.

professional boundary: These are the early childhood ethical, legal, and organizational structures for working in a profession. In early childhood, boundaries are guided by the NAEYC Code of Ethical Conduct.

professional identity: Our attitudes, values, knowledge, beliefs, and skills, framed by our Code of Ethics and enacted at the individual level in our professional practice.

professionalism: A shared set of professional values that guide the actions of a profession and its practice.

professional self-care: The strategies that you use for reflection, emotional supports, and professional skill development to assure that you are healthy and have resources and boundaries in early childhood settings.

professional skills: Tools to help navigate the "how-to" of our work. These are the professional competencies we need to understand children's development, support their learning, and guide their behaviors.

psychological well-being: A form of well-being that encompasses a holistic and positive approach to mental health, emphasizing the importance of positive emotions, relationships, and personal growth.

resource: Any tool, person, skill, disposition, or knowledge that assists an individual in life. Examples of resources include money, time, emotional intelligence, family members, and an engaged community.

self-awareness: The ability to identify and evaluate one's own emotions and psychological and behavioral responses. Self-awareness includes an awareness of strengths and limitations as well as an openness to learn from social interactions.

self-care: The practices of proactively caring for one's physical, social, cognitive, emotional, psychological, and spiritual well-being.

self-compassion: The practice of acknowledging one's own determined yet imperfect process of being the best one can be in work and in life.

self-criticize: To be hard on oneself in one's mental evaluation.

self-regulation: The process of regulating emotions by being flexible and coping with change. Self-regulation includes one's ability to stay regulated when emotions are high in oneself or others and one's ability to take responsibility for their emotions and their impact on others.

self-stewardship: The ability to lead one's physical, emotional, cognitive, social, psychological, and spiritual self in ways that actively promote and sustain well-being.

social skills: The tools for navigating interactions with others. Social skills include the ability to apply and interpret one's own emotions and those of others, use complex emotional vocabularies to convey a wide variety of emotions, practice active listening, and develop relationships.

social support system: The interwoven resources—including reflective, emotional, and skills-based supports—that a person has access to across social networks.

social well-being: A form of well-being that focuses on relationships and the roles they play in our lives.

somatic symptom: An indicator of stress that is physical, such as a headache, a stomach issue, and so on.

spiritual well-being: The aspect of well-being that focuses on our ability to discover meaning and purpose in our lives.

stress: A physical and mental reaction to difficult situations. Demands placed on the body from physically, mentally, and cognitively challenging situations create stress.

technical problem: A readily identifiable issue that can be quickly solved with concrete solutions, using existing expertise. Teachers learn how to solve technical problems through training, experience, and observing others.

trauma: A distressing, disturbing event or experience occurring once, multiple times, or repetitively over time that has an adverse effect on one's ability to function. Traumatic experiences are deeply difficult and emotionally challenging or draining; they often continue to have a negative effect on an individual after the event is over.

universal emotions: The shared emotions of the human experience, including anger, disgust, fear, happiness, sadness, and surprise; these are sometimes called basic emotions.

well-being: A positive sense of self that allows individuals to lead happy, productive lives and form and maintain healthy relationships.

wellness: An active process for pursuing well-being, which includes awareness and making choices that drive actions toward successful living.

whole self: All the aspects and domains of the self, including the physical, emotional, cognitive, social, psychological, and spiritual components.

References

Baumgartner, J., and J. Anderson. 2021. "The Self-Care Problem-Solving Pathway" Poster presented at the 2021 Annual Conference of the National Association for Early Childhood Teacher Educators (NAECTE). Orlando, FL, June 14.

Bronfenbrenner, U. 2005. "Ecological Systems Theory (1992)." In *Making Human Beings Human: Bioecological Perspectives on Human Development*, edited by U. Bronfenbrenner, 106–73. Thousand Oaks, CA: Sage Publications.

Brown, E. L., C. K. Vesely, D. Mahatmya, and K. J. Visconti. 2018. "Emotions Matter: The Moderating Role of Emotional Labour on Preschool Teacher and Children Interactions." *Early Child Development and Care* 188 (12): 1773–87.

Cannon, W. B. 1915. *Bodily Changes in Pain, Hunger, Fear, and Rage*. D. Appleton and Company.

de Schipper, E. J., J. M. Riksen-Walraven, S. A. Geurts, and C. de Weerth. 2009. "Cortisol Levels of Caregivers in Child Care Centers as Related to the Quality of Their Caregiving." *Early Childhood Research Quarterly* 24 (1): 55–63.

Folkman, S., R. S. Lazarus, R. J. Gruen, and A. DeLongis. 1986. "Appraisal, Coping, Health Status, and Psychological Symptoms." *Journal of Personality and Social Psychology* 50 (3): 571.

Gokalp, G. 2012. "Effects of Stress on Teacher Decision Making." In *International Perspectives on Teacher Stress,* edited by C. J. McCarthy, R. G. Lambert, and A. Ullrich, 69–94. Charlotte, NC: Information Age Publishing.

Heifetz, R. A., and D. L. Laurie. 1997. "The Work of Leadership." *Harvard Business Review* 75 (1): 124–34.

Hettler, B. 1976. *The Six Dimensions of Wellness Model.* Stevens Point, WI: National Wellness Institute.

Jeon, L., C. K. Buettner, and A. A. Grant. 2018. "Early Childhood Teachers' Psychological Well-Being: Exploring Potential Predictors of Depression, Stress, and Emotional Exhaustion." *Early Education and Development* 29 (1): 53–69.

J. Flowers Health Institute. n.d. "Eight Dimensions of Wellness." Accessed June 30, 2023. https://jflowershealth.com/8-dimensions-of-wellness.

Langford, R. 2006. "Discourses of the Good Early Childhood Educator in Professional Training: Reproducing Marginality or Working toward Social Change." *International Journal of Educational Policy, Research, and Practice: Reconceptualizing Childhood Studies* 7 (1): 115–25.

Lazarus, R. S., and S. Folkman. 1987. "Transactional Theory and Research on Emotions and Coping." *European Journal of Personality* 1 (3): 141–69.

Myers, J. E., and T. J. Sweeney. 2004. "The Indivisible Self: An Evidence-Based Model of Wellness." *The Journal of Individual Psychology* 60 (3): 234–44. https://core.ac.uk /download/pdf/149232976.pdf.

Myers, J. E., T. J. Sweeney, and J. M. Witmer. 2000. "The Wheel of Wellness Counseling for Wellness: A Holistic Model for Treatment Planning." *Journal of Counseling and Development* 78 (3): 251–66.

NAEYC (National Association for the Education of Young Children). 2011. NAEYC Code of Ethical Conduct and Statement of Commitment. Washington, DC: NAEYC. www.naeyc.org/sites/default/files/globally-shared/downloads/PDFs/resources /position-statements/Ethics%20Position%20Statement2011_09202013update.pdf.

———. 2022. *Developmentally Appropriate Practice in Early Childhood Programs Serving Children from Birth through Age 8*. 4th ed. Edited by Susan Friedman, Brian L. Wright, Marie L. Masterson, Barbara Willer, and Sue Bredekamp. Washington, DC: NAEYC.

National Institutes of Health. 2022. "Emotional Wellness Toolkit." Last reviewed August 8, 2022. https://www.nih.gov/health-information/emotional-wellness-toolkit.

National Wellness Institute. n.d. "The Six Dimensions of Wellness." National Wellness Institute. Accessed June 16, 2023. https://members.nationalwellness.org/page /Six_Dimensions.

Osgood, J. 2012. *Narratives from the Nursery: Negotiating Professional Identities in Early Childhood.* New York: Routledge.

Oxford University Press. 2018. S.v. "barrier." Updated May 18. https://www.encyclopedia .com/literature-and-arts/art-and-architecture/architecture/barrier.

Rath, T., and J. K . Harter. 2010. *Wellbeing: The Five Essential Elements*. New York: Simon and Schuster.

Taggart, G. 2019. "Early Childhood Education: From Maternal Care to Social Compassion." In *Compassion and Empathy in Educational Contexts*, edited by G. Barton and S. Garvis, 213–30. London: Palgrave Macmillan.

University of New Hampshire. n.d. *Emotional Wellness.* Accessed June 30, 2023. www.unh.edu /health/emotional-wellness.

Yosso, T. J. 2005. "Whose Culture Has Capital? A Critical Race Theory Discussion of Community Cultural Wealth." *Race, Ethnicity and Education* 8 (1): 69–91.